HOW TO QUICKLY IMPROVE MEMORY AND LEARNING

FOR KINESTHETIC LEFT AND RIGHT BRAIN SUPERLINKS LEARNING STYLES AND ADHD

RICKI LINKSMAN

HOW TO QUICKLY IMPROVE MEMORY AND LEARNING
FOR KINESTHETIC LEFT AND RIGHT BRAIN SUPERLINKS LEARNING STYLES AND ADHD

HOW TO QUICKLY IMPROVE MEMORY AND
LEARNING FOR KINESTHETIC LEFT AND RIGHT
BRAIN SUPERLINKS LEARNING STYLES AND ADHD
Copyright © 1993-2016 Ricki Linksman

This edition published 2016 by
National Reading Diagnostics Institute,
Naperville, Illinois

ISBN: 978-1-928997-46-7

© All rights reserved. No part of this book may be used
or reproduced in any manner whatsoever, whether print,
electronic, digital, or on the Internet, or in any format to be
invented in the future, without written permission
of the author.

Praise for Ricki Linksman's Books and Brain-Based Learning Methods

From Publications:

From "Woman News," New York, New York:
"There is a way to learn anything you want rapidly and successfully. The technique can be applied to any sort of learning in any field you choose. Each of us has a Superlink—the easiest method for us to fully learn information. Once you've found your Superlink, you can use it to learn in ways that are easy, effortless, and automatic." —published in an article in New York's "Woman News" called, "Mind Power: Smarten Up! Tap into Your Brain's Superlink—Learning Becomes Easy, Effortless, and Automatic"

From "L.A. Parent" and "San Diego Parent," California:
"All children in California will be reading at grade level or above by the end of third grade.' With this promise, California state leaders have made reading instruction in the early grades (K through Grade 3) a top priority in the public schools. So while the politicians are trying to do their part, how can parents help their little readers measure up? According to Ricki Linksman, author of *Your Child Can Be a Great Reader*, parents should first figure out their child's learning style. "Research shows that each of us receives information in different ways. Visual learners learn best through their eyes, auditory learners through their ears, tactile learners by touching, and kinesthetic learners by moving around."
–From an article in the "L.A. Times" and "San Diego Times," called "What is Your Child's Reading Style? If You Know How Your Child Reads You Can Help Him/Her Learn," by Judy Molland

Family Time Magazine:
Feb. 2007, published an article about how Keys to Reading Success™ helped two local suburban Chicago area schools (Fairmont and East Aurora) meet state standards.

From the Iowa "Gazette," Cedar Rapids, Iowa:
"Author Ricki Linksman has plenty of tips for parents who want to be sure their kids love to read, and can read well."

From the "Abilene Reporter-News," Abilene, Texas:
"This step-by-step guide is designed to help children overcome every kind of reading problem and get back up to grade level or beyond. It is filled with short, fun activities to do at home and provides pointers to boost self-esteem and motivation." (Jan. 24, 1999)

From Educators:
___

From a Public School District Superintendent:
"Ricki Linksman has synthesized the educational research into concepts which makes learning accessible to anyone. While the term differentiation of instruction is very popular in the world of education, Ricki Linksman provides concrete examples and techniques of combining learning styles with brain hemispheric preference to create an individualized "superlink." These techniques are personalized to open the pathways for anyone to learn anything quickly. For example, our junior high school went from 2/3 of the students below state level on state reading assessment tests to 2/3 of the students above state level in reading within eight months."
–Dr. Michael Early, Public School District Superintendent, Illinois, and former School Principal in West Suburban Chicago

From a School Superintendent:
"This is the only reading program I have found with the scientifically-based reading research that has proven statistics to raise reading levels so rapidly. Keys to Reading Success™ helped our school get off the state watch list that it had been on for 6 years, and this year—2006—we have finally made AYP or met state reading standards by using the program for only 6 months. The discipline problems in our school have been dramatically reduced as students went from reading below grade level to reading above grade level within 6 months. They are engaged in learning and have raised their self-esteem and motivation to achieve in school. Its parent involvement lessons in all learning styles and brain styles allow parents and teachers to work as a team for every child's success. This program ensures that every student can raise reading levels and test scores by Keys to Reading Success's™ comprehensive but easy-to-use reading diagnosis, learning styles and brain styles assessment, and its powerful, effective, and engaging teacher reading lesson plans in all learning styles. Using learning styles has helped every student learn to read in his or her most effective and fastest learning style possible."

–Dr. Doris Langon, Superintendent,
Fairmont District 89, Lockport, Illinois.

From a District School Superintendent on Gains in High School, Middle School, and Elementary School, including Indian Oaks Academy for Special Needs:
"Through using this program, significant gains were made in our district in elementary, middle, and high school on the CTBS (Cognitive Test of Basic Skills) test. Our ISAT (Illinois Standards Achievement Test) scores in reading showed significant growth. Gains in reading ranged from 1-8 grade levels in 9 months in the elementary, middle, and high school grades. From 86%-99% of students in grades 1-5 accelerated

to read from 1-8 years above grade level in reading within 9 months (including Regular Ed and Special Ed students). In the middle school, students rose from 1-6 years above grade level. In the high school 99.5% of students grades 9-12 rose from 1-2 grade levels in reading in 9 months."
 –M.S., Asst. Supt. Curriculum, Manteno School District

From a Principal of a Charter School in East Los Angeles, California:
"East Los Angeles school, Culture and Language Academy of Success (CLAS), a charter school devoted to African-American culture in the Los Angeles Unified School District rose from not meeting State Standards in reading to exceeding state standards in reading in 1 year using Ricki Linksman's *Keys to Reading Success* program using the techniques in *How to Learn Anything Quickly*. On a scale from 200-1000, they reached 773, with 35 points gain, and came close to the 800 superior school status. LA Unified District only reached 600 with a 9 point gain in 1 year. CLAS achieved 773, while California's state average was 635."
 –Principal, Dr. Sharroky Hollie,
 CLAS Charter School, Los Angeles, California

From a School Principal at Dieterich School in District 131, East Aurora, Illinois:
"With 83% of the school population speaking only Spanish and being enrolled in the English Language Learners (ELL) program, Dieterich School in East Aurora, Illinois, scored as the third highest in the district in their reading scores on the March 2006 ISAT Illinois State Achievement Test) reading test using Keys to Reading Success™ and Superlinks to Accelerated Learning™, using techniques from *How to Learn Anything Quickly*."
 –Principal, Dieterich Elementary School,
 East Aurora, Illinois

From an Elementary School:
"2/3 of the students in grades 1-3 rose from 1-7 grade levels in reading above grade level in one school year."
    –M.S., Teacher, Elementary School in Joliet, Illinois

From a Technology Director:
"We need to get past the assembly line way we teach and test. Through the use of technology and the Keys to Reading Success program, teachers can easily manage "progressive monitoring," diagnostic testing and reporting for students on an individual basis. This in turn allows teachers to customize each student's learning needs...what could be better?"
    -Vicki Dewitt, Technology Hub Director,
    Edwardsville, Illinois

From Learning Identity, South Africa:
"Ricki Linksman has a heart to make a difference in the lives of those who struggle with reading. She has developed a unique learning and reading program based on brain processing and learning styles, which undertakes to teach ANYONE how to read and learn and most importantly how to comprehend the content matter. We have had remarkable success with 100's of students utilizing Ricki's Keys to Reading Success and Superlinks to Accelerated Learning program, and consider it an honor to be a part of her work."
    –Trish Gatland, Learning Identity, South Africa

From Sports Coaches and Trainers:

From a Head Football Coach:
"Using these accelerated learning techniques such as teaching through learning styles has helped our university football team have its first winning season ever. The athletes learned

the plays faster and better through these techniques. We also had our best academic year ever, for our academic support to our athletes."

    –**Ken Karcher, University Head Football Coach**

From a Graduate of the National Academy of Sports Medicine (NASM) Certified Personal Trainer program:
"I passed the National Academy of Sports Medicine (NASM) Certified Personal Trainer (CPT) exam. The NASM CPT is considered the Cadillac of certifications for Personal Fitness Trainers and the exam has a notoriously high failure rate. The course itself (almost all correspondence based) is exceptionally detailed oriented and requires students to learn everything from intricate human anatomy to psychology, and everything in between. If I had known how hard it was going to be when I set out to do it, I don't think I would have even attempted it! While not all certifications are equal, those who have done the NASM CPT course and passed are in my opinion, border level scientists. Having done it myself, my respect level has gone through the roof not just for other NASM Certified Personal Trainers but also for myself. I wanted to let you know how grateful I am to you for all you did for me in learning about myself, my learning style (highly kinesthetic) and how to work around potential roadblocks. I have since learned even more about what makes me "tick." It's an exciting journey! Ricki, I wanted to take the time out to thank you from the bottom of my heart for everything you did for me--I don't think any of my success would have been possible without your help and expertise."

    –**Skye Middleton, NASM Certified Personal Trainer**

From Teachers Who Took the Master's Degree Teacher Education Superlinks Courses:

"In that one year, I learned more about teaching reading than from my entire college education."
　　　　　－M.S., Teacher, Farragut Elementary School, Joliet, Illinois

"The teacher training in reading is the best I have ever taken."
　　　　　－Special Education Teacher, Naperville Consolidated School District #203, Illinois

"The course in how to teach reading stretched my thinking about learning. The material was practical, hands-on, and relevant. Excellent trainer. It is the best course I have taken in years."
　　　　　－High School Title 1 Reading Teacher, Downers South High School, Downers Grove, Illinois

"I now have some tools and tests to evaluate why some of my students are not learning and to have techniques to teach to all my students. I recommend that every teacher take this training--it will open your eyes and hearts."
　　　　　－Teacher, Aurora Public Schools, Illinois

From Adult Learners:

"I am 26 years old and throughout my school career was labeled dyslexic. I never learned to read and ended up with a job and career that did not interest me. I wanted to go to college. Within 6 months of using Ricki Linksman's accelerated learning techniques, I learned to read well enough to pass the college entrance examination, and have been admitted to a college that will prepare me for the career I want."

–A.L., Chicago

"I am in my 50's and could never read. Through the Superlinks learning style and brain style test, I discovered that I had never been able to learn to read before because the method used in the school when I was growing up did not match the way I needed to learn. Working with Ricki Linksman and her accelerated learning techniques, I learned how to read in my best learning style and I can now enjoy books. Ricki then donated her services for free to our local branch of the *Literacy Volunteer of America* to train tutors in her Keys to Reading Success™ reading comprehension and memory program so they could keep working with adults who wanted to learn to read."

–J.S., Chicago

I had purchased Ricki's earlier book, *How to Learn Anything Quickly: Quick, Easy Tips to Improve Memory, Reading Comprehension, Test-Taking Skills, and Learning through the Brain's Fastest Superlinks Learning Style* a year ago when I was starting a study-at-home Medical Transcription program. At first, I somehow did not get past the first two pages. It ended up tucked in the bottom of my nightstand drawer. (I am a tactile-mixed with left-side dominate learner). Three weeks ago after struggling with comprehension and memory, I bit the bullet and got an extension. But, more importantly, I decided to commit to reading the book. Wow, I am glad I picked it up and forced myself to push past the first few pages. I have not been able to put it down, and will be finishing it up today. It was a really eye opening to see that the teaching styles of my teachers varied in my primary, elementary, high school, and college experiences. I passed Biology and Psychology with flying colors, but could not seem to get a passing grade from Nutrition class. Of course with your confidence shattered, you never see the parallels. You never look at the classes you did pass and wonder what went wrong; you just give up. (Or label yourself). How sobering to know that it was not my lack of ability; it was the learning style in which the information was presented—that each teacher had his or her own way of presenting the material, and it was the teachers that taught closer to my learning style where I excelled the most. I have a renewed commitment to complete my at-home study course and will take all that I have learned in this book with me throughout my life, for every subject I wish to learn. I have also bought two more copies for my husband and sister. This letter is just a huge thank you for writing such an easy to understand book, full of knowledge that can change anyone who is curious how to improve their learning and memory. Thank you!

-D.H., **adult learner**

From a Title 1 Success Story:
A 1st grader was not reading on level by mid-first grade. The parents and teachers were so concerned that they wanted to do an evaluation to see if he had a learning disability. During the waiting period for his evaluation, the Keys to Reading Success Accelerated Phonics Program was used with him in his Title 1 class. It was discovered that he was a kinesthetic learner. He used the kinesthetic component of the Keys to Reading Success Accelerated Phonics Program, and within months, mastered all the phonetic patterns and was not only able to read well at a 1st grade level, but accelerated into 2nd grade level reading, while still a first grader. By the time he was

evaluated by the psychologist, they discovered he actually had an I.Q. in the 140's and he was then placed in a gifted program. Had we not discovered his learning style and taught him through that method, he may have fallen even further behind in his reading level and it may have taken years to find out that he did not have a learning disability.

From University Instructors:
"Every teacher should use Keys to Reading Success. It is the most complete program of reading available. It is an excellent training tool for new teachers."
—**College Instructor for Graduate Education Courses for Teachers, Benedictine University, Lisle, Illinois**

From Parents Who Used the Superlinks Methods with Their Children and Teens:
"My high school son was getting D's and F's, but after a reading diagnosis and learning style assessment from Keys to Reading Success and receiving instruction in study skills and memory skills in his learning style, he is now getting A's. The program has also helped him on his SATs and ACTs."

—**M.O., Parent, Naperville, Illinois**

"When we started coming to Ricki Linksman at National Reading Diagnostics Institute, my son was in first grade, but reading at a kindergarten level, and his self-confidence was down. After working with Ricki for the past 11 months using her Keys to Reading Success™, Superlinks to Accelerated Learning™, and Off the Wall Phonics™ program, his reading level has improved so much that he is wanting to read books and complete Accelerated Reader™ book tests at school. My son is enjoying reading now that he reads at grade level and we will continue to work with Ricki to get him past grade level.

What a difference! Even his teacher in school has noticed and commented, 'He is to be commended for reading and taking tests on 23 books this quarter! He's starting to enjoy reading, which is wonderful.'"
–L.M., Wheaton Christian Grammar School,
Winfield, Illinois

"My child has made tremendous gains in a short time. His self-esteem has risen dramatically."
–A.P, Parent, Naperville

"My 10th grade son went from grades of 'F's" and 'D's' to 'A's' in 4 weeks. His study skills, comprehension, and memory has improved tremendously."
–Parent, Westmont

"In 6 months, my 4th grade child, who was reading 3 years below level, came up to grade level and is doing well in school."
–Parent, Lisle

"I have learned so much about how to help my son and about learning styles in general. I have to say that the frustration level when doing homework or reading has gone down dramatically.
–M.H., Chicago

"We have seen improved results in my son's tests and overall academics. In fact, he made the honor roll!! I appreciate the fact she is able to see how he best comprehends his reading material and incorporates the best plan for him. We are very happy to see his overall comprehension improve and especially his confidence. Thank you Ricki!"
–L.Z., parent

"My kindergartener is now reading 3rd grade books, and doing addition, subtraction, multiplication, and division over several months' time."
–Mr. R.M., Parent, Naperville

"For the first time, my 2nd grader could read on his grade level, and his self-esteem has increased tremendously."
–Parent, Chicago

"We wanted our 4-year-old child to qualify for a gifted school but she didn't achieve the necessary score on her first test. Within less than a year, she not only learned to read at a 3rd grade level, but was able to qualify for the gifted school. We are so thrilled with the results."
–S.D., Parent, Wheaton

"I home school my children and I learned how to accelerate their reading at home."
–Parent, Batavia

"My gifted child loves the challenging activities."
–Parent, Downers Grove

"I've looked for years for help for my son and Ricki Linksman is the only person that came through. My son has made more progress in these last 8 months than he has K through 6th grade. She provides concrete solutions to his specific areas that he needs help in. I recommend Ricki's book to anyone whose child is struggling at school or who wants to give their child an advantage to succeed. Ricki has not only helped my son to learn but his attitude and confidence has increased dramatically. I have seen amazing results for my son. Not only has his reading level improved dramatically but his confidence and enthusiasm are through the roof!"
–S.S, Parent, Illinois

"If you are reading this, you are probably concerned about the progress your child or grandchild is making in learning to read. I was in the same position several years ago. My grandson wasn't learning to read in his school. He had been left back in the same grade twice because he could not read. He was diagnosed with ADD and a learning disability. We spent years trying to find out why he could not read because he was a bright boy. As a concerned parent or grandparent, I got on the Internet and found Ricki Linksman's National Reading Diagnostics Institute and its Keys to Reading Success® and its Superlinks to Accelerated Learning™ programs which determined what his learning style and brain hemispheric preference was. The assessment determined he was a kinesthetic and tactile learner with a right brain hemispheric preference. It gave us a prescriptive plan to solve the problem and lessons in his best learning style. Within the first lesson of Keys to Reading Success®, using kinesthetic right brain learning techniques, my grandson read for the first time in his life, to his joy and excitement. After only one session with the Keys to Reading Success® materials, I watched this little guy read solid first-grade material that he had never been able to read before for the first time in his life. Yet, several hours before that first session, he had not even known the letters of the alphabet. I almost fell out of my chair, I was so excited. I knew then that I was on the right track, and I had found the right person and right techniques and program to teach this young lad how to read. He has been reading ever since. Within a few months, he was able to read at his grade level, and we were able to take him off his ADD medication. We now know what works for him and we attributed it to National Reading Diagnostics Institute and Keys to Reading Success. The developer of Keys to Reading Success®, Ricki Linksman, is truly the Michael Jordan of reading."

–**Rusty Acree, Concerned Grandparent, Retd. Naval Officer, and Field Judge for University Football Games, Richmond, Virginia**

And from his grandson, who wrote: When asked about what he liked best about his trip to Chicago, the lad wrote: "Learning to read. Thank you, Mrs. Linksman."

"Our teenager did not score well on the practice test for a high school entrance exam to Benet Academy, a college preparatory school. After a few months of work at National Reading Diagnostics Institute, areas of need were targeted and our teen got 99% on the actual entrance exam and was admitted to the preparatory school."
–Parent, Lisle

"Our son was in special education classes since 1st grade and by 7th grade still had not learned to read. We brought him to Ricki Linksman for a reading diagnosis and she gave him a Keys to Reading Success® reading diagnostic test, Superlinks™ learning style and brain style test, and tutoring instruction. Our son learned to read in months and no longer needed to be in special education. His self-esteem has gone up and he is so happy now."
–B. Burke., Parent, Miami, Florida

"My high school sophomore never dropped below A's or B's before, so when he dropped to a C in English, we were beside ourselves with frustration. After using these strategies for only 6 weeks, he not only went back up to A, but was the only student in the class to receive a writing award!"
–M.H., Parent

"We did not feel our middle school son had the skills to be ready for high school. He was struggling in many of his school subjects and even needed audios to read his assigned books to him. After only two months using these strategies, he can now read by himself, and his grades have improved to the point where the principal and teachers are astounded by his amazing progress! He feels proud of himself, enjoys school now, and has boosted his vocabulary, memory, study skills, and test-taking skills. The best part is that he does not need to be read to, but can read at and above his grade level all by himself!

–K.A, **Parent**

"My daughter struggled with reading in early elementary school, and I realized that when she read to me, she was only memorizing the book and could not read on her own. Ricki Linksman at National Reading Diagnostics Institute gave the Superlinks test and found out she was a kinesthetic right brain learner and the techniques in her school were not matching how she best learned. By using kinesthetic right brain techniques for her learning. Ricki not only taught her to read at grade level within a few months, but raised her several years above her age as well. Throughout the rest of her school career, she became a top reader and student in her class, no longer needed tutoring, and ended up in honors classes. In high school, she was number eleven in overall standing in her school. She returned to National Reading Diagnostics Institute to work with Ricki Linksman for ACT test prep, in her kinesthetic right brain learning style, and got a perfect score on the English ACT! She not only gained admission to numerous universities, but she was offered several scholarships, won academic awards, and ended up selecting a college, whose scholarship is paying $25,000.00 a year for each of the four years for her tuition. We are so glad we found National Reading Diagnostics Institute and Ricki Linksman and recommend her to any parent who wants to lay the foundation early for their child's future success in high school, college, and in life."

–J.O., **Parent, Wheaton, Illinois**

Awards and Achievements:

IASCD (Illinois Association for Supervision and Curriculum Development) awarded a WINN Research Certificate of Award of Merit for Outstanding Research to Ricki Linksman, Developer of Keys to Reading Success, for "Maximizing Reading Growth in Nine Months from 2-5 Grade Levels by Using Accelerated Phonics Taught through Learning Styles."

OTHER BOOKS AND RESOURCES BY THE AUTHOR, RICKI LINKSMAN

Books, ebooks, and Software about the Brain; Memory Improvement; Accelerated Learning through Learning Styles and Brain Styles; Kinesthetic, Tactile, Visual, Auditory Left and Right Brain Learners; Reading and Listening Comprehension Strategies; Accelerated Phonics; Vocabulary; Test-taking, Note-taking, and Study Skills and Test Prep for High School and College Entrance Exams, (ACT, SAT); Self-Esteem; Motivation; Concentration; and Focus

How to Learn Anything Quickly: Quick, Easy Tips to Improve Memory, Reading Comprehension, Test-Taking Skills, and Learning through the Brain's Fastest Superlinks Learning Style

How to Improve Memory Quickly: Quick, Easy Tips to Improve Memory through the Brain's Fastest Superlinks Learning Style

The Fine Line between ADHD and Kinesthetic Learners: 197 Kinesthetic Activities to Quickly Improve Reading, Memory, and Learning in Just 10 Weeks: The Ultimate Parent Guide to ADD, ADHD, and Kinesthetic Learners

How to Improve Reading Comprehension Quickly by Knowing Your Personal Reading Comprehension Style: Quick, Easy Tips to Improve Comprehension through the Brain's Fastest Superlinks Learning Style

Solving Your Child's Reading Problem through the Brain's Fastest Learning Style

From ADHD or ADD to A's: Improve Reading, Memory, and Learning Quickly for Kinesthetic Learners

Your Child Can Be a Great Reader

Keys to Reading Success™: Internet Reading Program (includes Linksman Passage Reading Tests, Linksman Phonics Diagnostic Test, and Superlinks Assessment, plus 1000s of pages of reading lesson plans in all learning styles: Kinesthetic, Tactile, Visual, and Auditorywith adaptations for right and left brain learners in reading comprehension, phonics, vocabulary, test-taking strategies, test prep, and study skills.

Superlinks to Accelerated Learning Assessment™ (includes Linksman Learning Style Preference Assessment™ and Linksman Brain Hemispheric Preference Assessment™)

Off the Wall Phonics (Accelerated K-12, College, and Adult Phonics Program to Improve Reading Comprehension, Word Reading and Fluency for Kinesthetic, Tactile, Visual, and Auditory Learners, both Right brain and Left Brain Learners)

Kinesthetic Vocabulary Activities Your Child Will Love

Tactile Vocabulary Activities Your Child Will Love

How to Quickly Improve Memory and Learning for Kinesthetic Left and Right Brain Superlinks Learning Styles and ADHD

How to Quickly Improve Memory and Learning for Tactile Left and Right Brain Superlinks Learning Styles

How to Quickly Improve Memory and Learning for Visual Left and Right Brain Superlinks Learning Styles

How to Quickly Improve Memory and Learning for Auditory Left and Right Brain Superlinks Learning Styles

How to Quickly Improve Reading Comprehension for Kinesthetic Left and Right Brain Superlinks Learning Styles

How to Quickly Improve Reading Comprehension for Tactile Left and Right Brain Superlinks Learning Styles

How to Quickly Improve Reading Comprehension for Visual Left and Right Brain Superlinks Learning Styles

How to Quickly Improve Reading Comprehension for Auditory Left and Right Brain Superlinks Learning Styles

How to Quickly Improve Study, Note-taking and Test-taking Skills for Kinesthetic Left and Right Brain Superlinks Learning Styles

How to Quickly Improve Study, Note-taking and Test-taking Skills for Tactile Left and Right Brain Superlinks Learning Styles

How to Quickly Improve Study, Note-taking and Test-taking Skills for Visual Left and Right Brain Superlinks Learning Styles

How to Quickly Improve Study, Note-taking and Test-taking Skills for Auditory Left and Right Brain Superlinks Learning Styles

Vowel and Consonant Guide

Superlinks to Accelerated Learning: Phonics Diagnostic Test (Student Test Booklet and Instructional Manual)

For other products, books, eBooks, software, trainings, and e-courses visit:

www.readinginstruction.com
www.keyslearning.com
www.superlinkslearning.com
www.keystoreadingsuccesss.com
or e-mail: info@keyslearning.com

Special note to the reader: This book is part of a series. Other books in the series include: improving reading comprehension; and improving study, note-taking, and test-taking skills for learning any subject. If you want one book that contains all the books in the series combined in the full compendium than you can buy: ***How to Learn Anything Quickly: Quick, Easy Tips to Improve Memory, Reading Comprehension, and Test-taking Skills through the Brain's Fastest Superlinks Learning Style.*** If you wish a book focused on only one learning style for both left and right brain learners, the individual volumes for each learning style are available in this series.

Dedicated to

parents and teachers who devote their lives to helping their children or students, whether children, teen or adults, be all they can be in life.

Table of Contents

Praise for Ricki Linksman's Books and Brain-Based Learning Methods i

Other Books and Resources by the Author, Ricki Linksman xvii

Introduction 1

Chapter 1: What is a Kinesthetic Right and Left Brain Learner? 7

Chapter 2: How Kinesthetic Left Brain Learners Can Improve Memory to Learn Anything Quickly 11

Chapter 3: How Kinesthetic Right Brain Learners Can Improve Memory to Learn Anything Quickly 21

Chapter 4: Preparation and Planning for Kinesthetic Learners to Learn Anything Quickly 33

Chapter 5: Choosing a Kinesthetic Learner's Best Instruction, Materials, and Learning Environment to Improve Memory to Learn Anything Quickly 49

Chapter 6: Strategies to Improve a Kinesthetic Learner's Memory 61

Chapter 7: Applying What You Have Learned About Improving a Kinesthetic Learner's Memory and Learning 95

Appendix 99

Bonus for Readers 109

About the Author: Ricki Linksman 113

Contact Information 121

A Special Gift for Readers 123

INTRODUCTION

Unlock the key to your kinesthetic brain to increase your memory powers and remember *everything* you read.

Are you a kinesthetic learner who is frustrated because you have a hard time remembering what you read and hear at your job, in school, or in your daily life?

Do you feel restless if you have to sit still and need to get up and move a lot?

Do you like to compete, always needing to win, and become frustrated when you don't win?

When you do sit, do you tap your feet, wiggle your legs, and even sit partly out of your seat?

Do you feel you listen to people better when you are moving?

Do you wish you can have better recall of names of people, places, facts and figures unless it is related to sports or activities?

Have you or others thought your need to move is not due to a kinesthetic learning style but attributed to having ADHD or ADD?

Have you already been diagnosed with ADHD or ADD and do not really feel you are because your attention is great when you are moving or actively engaged in doing things you like?

Do you truly have ADHD or ADD but want techniques that will help you learn using your love of movement?

If you find any of these characteristics describe you, you may be a kinesthetic learner who learns best by moving your body and large motor muscles.

If you are a kinesthetic learner who feels that learning through only a visual, auditory, or tactile teaching style has been difficult, relax! You are not alone. This book will give you the secrets to your kinesthetic brain and unlock your best memory power!

Many kinesthetic learners have discovered that by moving when learning, they dramatically improved their ability to remember everything they read.

Many people who either suspected, or have been diagnosed, or just have similar characteristics to those with ADHD or ADD have benefitted from these kinesthetic memory techniques. In fact, many with ADHD or ADD who used these techniques have found them so successful that with their doctor's approval they have been able to reduce or eliminate medication because the kinesthetic memory techniques helped them. Of course, if under medical supervision, follow your doctor's advice regarding medication. With or without medication, you can supplement your therapy with kinesthetic memory techniques to help you achieve your learning goals.

You too can be a winner and master your memory capabilities by doing the simple techniques in this book.

How great would your life be if you could recall every book chapter or study guide you read? Imagine how successful you would be if you mastered your own memory! What would you do with the extra time you would save by not having to reread multiple times to remember text. Experience the confidence and raised self-esteem you would have when you could recall anything you choose to remember.

How to Quickly Improve Memory and Learning for Kinesthetic Left and Right Brain Superlinks Learning Styles contains easy practical exercises and activities for the kinesthetic left brain or right brain learner.

Over thirty years of applying brain research to improve memory, I have helped kinesthetic learners of all ages by teaching them these quick, easy, and fun tips, activities, exercises, and strategies in this book to achieve success in the shortest possible time. You can use them for yourself, or if a parent use them with your children or teens. If you are a teacher or instructor, you can use these methods with your kinesthetic students. Sports coaches and athletic trainers can teach their playbook to kinesthetic learners with these strategies. Employers can train kinesthetic employees to learn or master their job more easily. Professionals who need to communicate with kinesthetic clients, patients, or customers can better get your message across.

Develop the confidence to learn whether for school, college, job, career, sports, or hobbies. You do not have to wait for months or years to learn these secrets to learning and remembering quickly—they are available now within this book for the kinesthetic left brain or right brain learner to use to learn anything for any purpose.

While there are many memory books and courses on the market, this one has proven to work the fastest and easiest with proven measurable results because it is geared to how YOUR brain learns and remembers. Every one processes information differently and what works for one person may not work for you. This is the first program available that tailors the memory improvement and learning skills for how YOU learn best.

In this book written for kinesthetic learners, whether with a left brain or right brain preference or a combination of both, you hold quick, easy tips to increase your memory to learn anything quickly.

Use your brain's energy powers to succeed in the competitive job market, whether to get hired for a job, keep your job, or keep pace with new information and technology in a rapidly-changing job market. *How to Quickly Improve Memory and Learning for Kinesthetic Left and Right Brain Superlinks Learning Styles* gives you fast, simple, and powerful memory strategies to remember and comprehend *everything* you read and learn for rapid success.

It has been rewarding to receive feedback from people throughout the world describing how these easy methods to increase memory and learning has transformed their lives by helping them achieve success in any field—quickly.

My hope is that *How to Quickly Improve Memory and Learning for Kinesthetic Left and Right Brain Superlinks Learning Styles* unlocks your own amazing brain power and fills you with confidence and high self-esteem. Starting right now, may you experience the joys of learning as you achieve your life's goals.

–**Ricki Linksman**

Chapter 1:
What is a Kinesthetic Right and Left Brain Learner?

Do you want to increase your memory and improve learning techniques to learn any subject quickly? Are you a job seeker or employee looking for a new job and must remember new skills fast? Do you find it hard to keep up with change? Are constant innovations at your place of employment forcing you to spend time continually learning new skills or learning to use new technological equipment? Do you wish you had the memory power to learn the skills required at your job more rapidly?

Do you wish you could remember what you study and read? Do you feel that your test scores do not reflect the great amount of time you spend studying? Are you frustrated by the slow speed at which you learn? Do you feel so hopeless that you do not think you can learn much at all?

Take heart! You can successfully learn how to learn quickly anything you want. The purpose of this book is to give you fast, easy strategies to reach your learning goals quickly. This book gives the **kinesthetic left or right brain learner** a method to improve your memory successfully and quickly. It is user-friendly and simple to follow. It is written for everyone: for people of all ages, at all levels of education. It is designed to help the kinesthetic left or right brain learner learn quickly.

You will learn strategies and techniques to improve your memory that can be applied to any field you choose. Once you have improved your memory and learning techniques, you will be able to use these kinesthetic learning methods for the rest of your life for anything you wish to learn. This book for the kinesthetic left or right brain learner will help you find the path to accelerated learning—a study method of learning how to learn that works best for you.

Sit back and relax. Follow the fast, easy, and simple steps in the book and you will emerge from the last page of this book an expert on how *you* learn best and how to apply it to any field you want.

Kinesthetic learners require body movement and action for optimal results. They need to move around and use their muscles to learn. They learn through action, doing, exploration, and discovery.

Not all kinesthetic people are alike. Some like to learn by verbal instructions, and others become annoyed when anyone speaks when they are engaged in activity. They prefer instead nonverbal demonstration that they could copy. Some kinesthetic people like to talk about what they do, while others do not want to talk at all about the physical experiences in which they engaged.

After we use our learning style to comprehend information, our brain processes and stores the information either using the left side (left hemisphere) of the brain or the right side (right hemisphere). Each side has a different memory style, or its own way of thinking about and looking at the world. Some of us have a **left brain hemispheric preference** and some have a **right brain hemispheric preference**, while some use both sides of the brain. **Left brain learners** tend to be sequential and process information in a linear manner. **Right brain learners** tend to think globally, seeing the big picture, and connecting seemingly unrelated ideas. Also, left brain learners think more in symbols such as letters, words, and numbers, while right brain learners think more in sensory or graphic or pictorial images of sights, sounds, smell, tastes, touch, and movement, without words.

Chapter 2:
How Kinesthetic Left Brain Learners Can Improve Memory to Learn Anything Quickly

What Is a Kinesthetic Left Brain Learner?

Kinesthetic left brain learners learn quickly and can improve memory through movement and action of their body and large motor muscles in an organized, systematic way. Because the language function is in the left side of the brain, they can verbalize movement activities in systematic, structured ways.

Kinesthetic left brain learners need to move a great deal and are restless when they have to stay in one place. If they are forced to stay in one seat too long, they will begin to move or rock in the seat, kick their legs, or get out of the seat spontaneously. Others may be distracted by their movements. Yet if they are given an opportunity to use their body, they will actually stick to a task with great concentration; it is when they are denied movement that they find some other outlet for their kinesthetic needs that may not be productive. They are going to move anyway, whether they are restricted or not—so at least their lessons should be structured in a way that includes movement as a positive part of their training.

They like team sports, organized games, or exercises that

have rules and are done in a step-by-step way. Many kinesthetic left brain people are extremely coordinated and can time their movements to be in synch with others. They may excel in synchronous swimming, gymnastics, acrobatics, or choreographed dance.

Not all kinesthetic left brain people are athletic and coordinated, but they still require sequential movement activities in other fields, whether they are developing real estate, designing a software program or app, find a cure for a disease, or exploring a new hobby. Movement for them can be just mentally moving from one topic or project to another. They are systematic and orderly and tend to stick to and complete a task before moving on.

They need room to move around and comfortable sitting areas to stretch out and relax. If a place does not allow them to move about or has no action-oriented activity, kinesthetic left brain people will feel uncomfortable and bored because there is nothing for them to do there.

They enjoy talking with other people while in motion or physically doing something, such as jogging, exercising, or working with someone else.

How Kinesthetic Left Brain Learners Can Improve Memory to Learn Anything Quickly

Kinesthetic left brain learners can improve their memory to learn quickly by using an organized, systematic, step-by-step approach that involves moving their bodies and muscles. They are language-oriented, so they can describe what they are doing and follow verbal systematic directions for movement activities. They can get on an exercise bike and read or study while pedaling, or walk around the room while memorizing the lines to a play. Learning games, simulations, role-playing and competitions are great ways for them to learn. Whatever movement they do, they prefer to use a formula, structure, or outline for their work.

It may appear to others that kinesthetic left brain people are not listening because they are constantly moving, and they process thought better when their eyes are down and away from a speaker, but they are attentive when they are in motion. It is so stressful for them to sit still with their eyes on a speaker that they cannot concentrate on listening. Yet when they are moving about, they are relaxed, comfortable, and attentive.

Hands-on materials and manipulatives are important to kinesthetic learners, but they benefit more from moving their entire bodies, not just their hands. The simple act of standing up helps them learn because it gets their legs, arms, and other muscles moving. They need to write with large markers or chalk on a flip chart, white board, or chalkboard while standing. Doing math problems or outlining a report on a flip chart helps them to think better. By writing in large letters on a whiteboard, they can involve their arm muscles and the activity into the kinesthetic realm. Kinesthetic left brain people do not prefer to doodle or draw as tactile learners do, but they may do so only when it is the only movement they are permitted in a constrained work or learning situation. It offers them some movement of their arm and hands, which may not fully satisfy them but it is better than sitting still.

In whatever subject they learn, kinesthetic left brain learners need to learn by doing something in a sequential way. Just listening to lectures and verbal explanations is not enough for them to assimilate the material. They can benefit by volunteering to be a how-to demonstrator instead of just watching a demonstration. If they hear action words in sequential order, they will physically understand the material. They need a coach who will actively work through the steps of a process. If they are learning how to use a computer, they have to be at a computer while going through each step. If they are learning about carpentry, they will need the tools and materials so as the instructor models for them how to build something they can do it as they learn. They will remember not what an instructor does, but what *they* do.

When doing study skills or note taking to memorize material for a test or examination, they recall what they *did* with the material. If the subject is math or science, they need to work out the problems or experiments in a step-by-step way in real-life applications; for example, by doing the math required for sending a spaceship to the moon, mixing chemicals to produce medicine, or writing a software program. If circumstances do not allow a kinesthetic left brain learner to do an activity, their next best resort is to watch activity—movies on television or in a theater, using streaming video, or watching a program on the Internet or on any electronic device, preferably sequentially-presented programs.

Another kinesthetic method for them is to visualize themselves in their mind moving. In this way they can experience the action within themselves without being noticeable to others. They should feel in their mind that their body is moving or enacting whatever it is they are trying to learn, even while their physical body remains still. This will also activate neuronal growth in their brain as if they had actually physically performed the action.

Kinesthetic left brain learners thrive on achievement, winning, challenges, and discovery. Being goal-oriented, they enjoy the thrill of the game, and their motivation increases in a competitive environment. They like competing with themselves and beating their own record or against teams. Since the left side of the brain handles facts and figures, kinesthetic left brainers tend to discuss game scores or keep records of achievement of others or themselves. Converting any learning experience into a competitive game helps kinesthetic left brain people learn better.

Kinesthetic left brain learners need manipulatives; organized games; building materials; sports equipment, such as balls, basketball hoops, jump ropes, and exercise bikes; science projects; large markers to write on large pieces of paper, flip charts, or white boards; computers; musical instruments; hands-on models; kits; or real objects to move.

They like high action yet structured programs, games, and apps on the computer or any electronic digital device.

Kinesthetic left brain learners can read, work, or study with or without music. Moving or dancing to the rhythm and beat of music can stimulate them to work better. When their muscles are in motion, stress is reduced, their attention and motivation increase, and they learn faster. Kinesthetic left brain people enjoy playing musical instruments that engage the whole body. They can handle a systematic approach to learning an instrument and will attend to the technical aspects of playing, such as timing, rhythm, and reading music.

Working in cooperative groups or teams helps the kinesthetic left brain learner because they can move around from group to group. They like to work from a plan or structured outline, so they know each step of the process beforehand. Interaction with different people in different groups fulfills their need to be where the action is.

To improve memory to learn anything quickly, kinesthetic left brain learners should get actively involved in the reading material, either by physically acting out the text or imaging themselves doing so. They should imagine experiencing their muscles moving by acting out in their mind what the words describe in sequential order. To engage their interest and remember what they read, kinesthetic left brain learners need to convert the words into an action movie in their mind in which they are part of the action. They tend to forget whatever they do not imagine themselves "doing" in their mind as they read.

Kinesthetic left brain learners prefer to read action-packed books. They like to read about movement-oriented activities in a detailed, step-by-step, well-organized way if it can help them improve what they do. The left brain's ability to think in terms of language helps them understand verbal or written directions for action-oriented subjects. They enjoy "how-to" books that help them perform better if written in logical, sequential ways. Business people enjoy reading how-to suggestions for improving their businesses. Sports lovers enjoy books that help them perfect their techniques.

Kinesthetic left brain learners need a purpose and action-oriented reason to be motivated to read. If they know their sales will increase if they read the training manual, they will be sure to read it. If they know they need to pass the driver's license examination, they will force themselves to read the manual.

In the work place, kinesthetic left brain people can be found in jobs that require movement along with left brain organization, putting what they do into words, or giving detailed verbal directions to others. Jobs that require traveling, speaking, and being clear and organized in one's presentation are found in sales, marketing, district management, owning a self-employed business, teaching, and training. Kinesthetic left brain people who go into the sciences may be involved in experiments, research and laboratory work, or medical fields, becoming doctors and nurses.

Since they excel at movement jobs that are related to being

on time, a function of the left side of the brain, they may be pilots, train conductors, chauffeurs, truck drivers, delivery people, or parcel, express mail, or postal workers. Work that involves the physical body and using details, measurements, and precision are construction, engineering, roadwork, farming, painting, wallpapering, plumbing, electrical work, cleaning, furniture crafting, and doing repair work. Jobs that require physically protecting other people and that use the left brain attention to structure, organization, and rules are in areas such as the armed forces, such as in the Army, the Navy, the Coast Guard or the Marines, or in the police force, fire department, or secret service.

Kinesthetic left brain learners may be involved in organized sports and games or may use their verbal abilities to become sportscasters or coaches and instructors in movement fields such as aerobics, exercise, or dance. They may write action stories, sports columns, reviews of movies, dance, or theatrical performances, or organized and structured how-to books. Their ability to visualize action on a screen or stage may make them good screenwriters and playwrights. As artists, they are structured and systematic in their work and will portray detailed action through illustrations, cartoons, comic strips, or commercials for advertising. They may be directors of movies, plays, or dance groups. They may become actors and actresses, musicians, performers, or instructors of performing arts that require body movement.

Adapting Learning to a Kinesthetic Left Brain Learning Style

Kinesthetic left brain learners should ask instructors to let them do movement activities in a sequential way to learn the material. If instruction is presented as a lecture, they need to ask for outlines or study guides or do their own note taking in sequential order, so they can convert the words into: a) actions; b) a movie in their mind in which they imagine themselves doing the action; or c) an outline while they stand up and write it in large size on a flip chart or white board. They can find sequential material, either written and in audio-visual format that relates to the subject and convert the text into a physical action or an imagined action in their mind.

Chapter 3:
How Kinesthetic Right Brain Learners Can Improve Memory to Learn Anything Quickly

What Is a Kinesthetic Right Brain Learner?

Kinesthetic right brain learners can improve memory to learn quickly through moving their gross motor muscles in a creative, imaginative, free-flowing, and unstructured way. They do not think in words, but get information intuitively.

They become highly restless if forced to stay still or remain in one place too long. Kinesthetic right brain learners will feel so constrained and physically stressed that they will start to move around anyway. Their need to keep moving and changing activities may make they look hyperactive to others. It is actually when they are denied movement that they look distracted. It is better to give them movement activities related to the learning task, such as learning games, exercises, or simulations. They will then be able to concentrate as well as people of other styles do when working in their element. Unless given productive activities related to their work, they will kick or swing their legs under the table, drum on the tabletop, slouch, rock in their seats, or find excuses to get up, whether it is to get a snack or look out a window.

Not all kinesthetic right brain learners are athletes. There are many other activities that involve movement. For them, movement can be moving in their mind from one topic or project to another.

Kinesthetic right brain learners can think about several things simultaneously and can have many projects going on at once. They can keep each one straight in their minds without any difficulty. They work in an impulsive, quick way, wanting to see results immediately so they can move on to another activity. In the rush to complete a project, they may not worry about whether the parts were done to perfection. They see the whole picture, not the details.

There are times when they consider a job done just by having thought of it. Some kinesthetic right brain people put the idea out, do some preliminary work, and move on to another project. It is up to the detail-oriented people around them to pick up the pieces and complete the task so they can then move on to create new inventions. They have a wealth of new ideas and discoveries, like a brainstorm session in motion, giving the world a seeming endless supply of novel, unique ideas.

Being goal-oriented, kinesthetic right brain learners have the ability to get things done, handling many projects at once. They are not time-oriented, so they do not tend to stick to schedules, routines, or time constraints. They are go-with-the-flow people who will do what they feel like at the moment. They can keep work moving and be a wealth of creativity and imagination, although others have to be willing to accept their lack of consciousness of time. At work, as frequently as they arrive late, they may also become so absorbed in a task that they may stay overtime just to complete it, giving them more productivity than what they are paid to do!

A kinesthetic right brain learner needs a comfortable environment, full of activity, with room to stretch out and move. Some will get up and leave if they are bored or in a restricted environment. Being outdoors is high on their list because there they can move freely.

Kinesthetic right brain people enjoy being with other people when they can do something together that does not require a lot of talk. Watch them during a football game and you may hear grunts, moans, or cheers. They can communicate action without speaking and use their body and arms to dramatize or express what they want to describe. When they do talk, they use short action words and get to the point quickly.

How Kinesthetic Right Brain Learners Can Improve Memory to Learn Anything Quickly

Kinesthetic right brain people can improve their memory to learn quickly by moving in an unstructured, imaginative, and free-flowing way. They need to use their bodies and muscles to learn. Thus, they can learn better while cycling on a stationary bike, memorizing material by jumping rope, simulating or role-playing a situation, performing experiments, or playing creative games.

Kinesthetic right brain learners, often adventuresome and daring, enjoy challenges. This group just needs to jump in and "do it." They pick up the how-to information by intuition or gut feelings and learn by trial and error, exploration, and discovery. They fully grasp the overall patterns of any situation and know what to do. Their excellent visual-spatial relations, intuition, and quick reflexes enable them to look at a problem, instantaneously judge a situation, and move accordingly, without words or written directions, to find the solution.

Kinesthetic right brain learners do not require step-by-step, detailed instructions. They are whole-to-part learners who need to see the big picture or overview first and fill in the details later. For example, they will not give a detailed verbal account of a sports event—they will give the highlights and the winning score: the bottom line. If they see an entire math problem worked out with the answer and several examples, they can figure out how to solve similar problems.

Kinesthetic right brain learners listen better to others while in motion, with their eyes focused down and away from the speaker. They remember more when they are in motion than when they are sitting still. When they are moving, they can relax, concentrate, and absorb information better.

They learn better by standing up to work. Writing on a flip chart or whiteboard with large markers works better for them than writing while sitting. By involving their whole arm, legs, and body, they can put the activity into the kinesthetic realm. Making a mind map of material they need to know by using their whole arm to write provides more activity and helps them recall what they learned. They doodle not because of a tactile need to write but because it offers more movement than sitting still.

They need active real-life or simulated experiences. For example, when learning about accounting they would prepare a budget for a real company or an imaginary one they created for this learning experience. If volunteers are needed for a demonstration, kinesthetic right brain learners jump at a chance to get out of their seats and do something. If they are learning a dance, they will remember it not by watching someone else do it, but by doing it themselves. They need to immerse themselves fully in the experience in an unstructured way. Many of them do not want long explanations; they want to figure something out for themselves. They need teachers who will take on the role of a coach, use only key action words, and guide them if they ask for help.

If a situation does not permit the kinesthetic right brain learner to do an activity, their next resort is to watch activity on television, DVDs, videos, or movies. To remember what they learn, they need to act out the material or visualize themselves dramatizing it as if a movie were playing in their head. When they visualize they need to feel the movement in their muscles. Their body may move and sway as they go through the movements in their mind. When they receive directions to drive to a friend's house, they experience themselves turning the car right or left, or whipping along the curve in the road in their mind.

Good learning materials for a kinesthetic right brain learner are manipulatives, games, building materials, tools, sports equipment, balls, exercise bikes, large flip charts, whiteboards, large markers, computers with action games, percussion instruments, guitars or organs, rhythmic music, hands-on models, or real objects to move. They like unstructured, nonsequential, high-action, fast-moving video games, apps, and interactive programs. If a computer program is too slow or too structured, they become bored. They prefer moving a mouse, joystick, or swiping their fingers across a screen rather than using keystrokes on a keyboard.

Competitions and challenges interest kinesthetic right brain people, either in games or on the job. They may participate in contests that determine who can sell or produce the most. They are goal-oriented and enjoy the thrill of winning points for themselves or their team. Make a game of anything and they will learn it.

Kinesthetic right brain learners do better using note-taking, study skills and test-taking strategies by remembering what action they *did* while learning. For them to concentrate, distractions caused by the movement of others have to be eliminated. Working in a study carrel, using a divider, or facing a wall can keep them from noticing the movement of others, but they have to be comfortable while studying. Being stretched out on the floor or couch gives their muscles freedom of movement. They can work and study with or without music. Because they do not listen to the words, music does not interfere with their reading. The rhythm or beat stimulates their muscles to move or dance in time to the music. Their stress is reduced and their attention and motivation increases.

By working in cooperative groups, kinesthetic right brain learners have an opportunity to move around more from group to group. They thrive on change and on interacting with different people to satisfy their need for action.

To improve memory, kinesthetic right brain learners need to convert words into a movie in which they are part of the action. Imagining that they are the director of a movie and converting the book or script into action scenes, while describing the action that would appear on their movie screen, will make a book come alive for them. Whatever they do not feel themselves doing—or imagining they are doing—as they read will be lost to their memory.

They read for the main idea or big picture, skipping small details, and are impatient with too many words. Thus, they tend to miss reading comprehension questions that deal with details, time sequence, or abstract ideas. It is not that they cannot remember the details, but they need kinesthetic right brain techniques to master them.

Kinesthetic right brain learners prefer short or highly

action-packed books or how-to books that help them perform better. Unlike their left brain counterparts, they need diagrams, photographs, or illustrations. They do not like to read a book from cover to cover but tend to skip around, getting what they need from it. They may learn by just looking at the pictures, glancing at the captions, or flipping through the pages, catching stray sentences that may give them all they need to know about a topic. They have an intuitive sense that helps them find what they need.

Kinesthetic right brain learners need to know the end product before they start. Thus, they need to know the reason they are reading something. They will be motivated if they feel it will help them do something better. Watch them zip through a book if they feel it will help them be the top in their field, boost their sales, or get a promotion. Books with summaries or key points at the beginning or end of the chapter help them find what is important and relevant to them.

In the workforce, kinesthetic right brain people can be found in jobs that require movement and frequent change. They may not attend to details, but they will work quickly to get a job done rapidly. With this group, speed and completion takes priority over spending a great deal of time on detail, as long as the end product works.

As scientists, kinesthetic right brain people enjoy inventing, doing research and laboratory work, or experimenting in the fields of paleontology, anthropology, quantum physics, or chemistry. If they go into medicine, they may run their own practices so they can have the freedom to set their own hours, or move from one patient to another in ten different rooms.

They may be involved in sports fields, as athletes, coaches, instructors, trainers, or owning a sports facility or team. They may be involved with dancing, gymnastics, golf, track, skiing, skating, swimming, sailing, snorkeling, surfing, biking, gymnastics, horseback riding, Rollerblading, karate, judo, horseback riding, or aerobics, and so on. They may play football, soccer, hockey, tennis, and basketball for fun, but may have to work harder to adjusting to being on an organized professional team because of the rigors of the schedule, discipline, and routine involved in that lifestyle.

They may enjoy the adventure and risks involved in police work, firefighting, the space program, or the Army, Navy, Marines, or Coast Guard. Many of them like to be self-employed so they do not have to follow someone else's schedule. They may run their own computer, construction, painting, wallpapering, cleaning, moving, lawn, maintenance, plumbing, electrical, or repair companies.

They can be involved in building, making, or fixing things such as cars, houses, boats, motorcycles, computers, appliances, machines, or furniture. They may do work that requires physical exertion such as construction, building bridges, or lifting boxes. Some work in jobs that require traveling, but with little talk. Long-distance driving, flying, chauffeuring, making deliveries, and trucking may satisfy their need to move, if they are not constrained by time schedules.

Kinesthetic right brain writers write short action stories that get to the point or how-to books that give key points without much detail. If they are artists, they like art requiring action—huge canvases or sculptures with strong movement of color and design. They tend to make quick, impressionistic drawings that give a general idea of what they are trying to say. If they are actors or actresses, they may prefer parts with less talk and more action or be stunt people. If they are musicians, they enjoy playing instruments in which they can move their body. If they are singers, they prefer doing so with movement or dance. Kinesthetic right brain learners tend to be better at playing by ear rather than reading notes. They also tend to be imaginative and can come up with new tunes or forms of music.

Their imagination, new ideas, openness to change, and inventiveness make them an excellent resource. Their commitment to "doing" makes them product oriented and able to produce a large amount of work in a short amount of time. As they move, the world also moves forward into new avenues and directions.

Adapting Learning to a Kinesthetic Right brain Style

Kinesthetic right brain learners need to ask their instructor to provide the big picture or overview using short, sensory language and let them do kinesthetic activities in a global, creative, free-flowing way. Since it is hard for kinesthetic right brain learners to follow auditory presentations, they need a written copy of the notes or readings or take dictation of a lecture and convert each word into: a) a movie in their mind in which they imagine and feel themselves acting out the parts; b) a drawing they make with key words or numbers in colorful, artistic, and creative ways, while standing up at a white board or flip chart and writing with their large arm muscles; c) a mind map in color in which they show the main topic, the details, and their interconnections; or d) a kinesthetic project. They may need to find corresponding pictures, movies, or activities, in which they can participate in real-life demonstrations. They can convert information into a mind map that gives the big picture of the subject they are learning.

Chapter 4:
Preparation and Planning for Kinesthetic Learners to Learn Anything Quickly

You are now ready to begin the process of accelerating learning. The first steps are to ask yourself the following questions before you get started:

- What is my motivation, purpose, or goal for learning this subject?
- What do I already know about this subject?
- What do I need to know about this subject?
- What is the best way for me to learn?
- How can I raise my self-esteem and use positive thinking about myself?
- What are some relaxation and stress reduction techniques to optimize learning?
- How can I visualize success?

What Is My Motivation, Purpose, or Goal for Learning This Subject?

People remember things that serve a purpose in their lives. Every day we are bombarded with information that we see, hear, smell, taste, or touch, but we only remember what we consider important; otherwise, we would be unable to sort through the multitude of stimuli we receive.

Our brain has the decision-making capacity to sort out what is relevant. Whatever it decides to remember, it will remember. This is a choice we make continually and it is something we should keep in mind when it comes to learning. As information is conveyed to us, we can observe it passively and let it bounce off us, or we can take it in and retain it. Think about several subjects you have learned throughout your life. Were there times when you attended a lecture or read a book, hearing and seeing the words, but moments later the information was gone? You did not really *learn* the material—you did not commit it to memory. Were there other times that you decided you really needed to remember the information you received so you paid closer attention to it, absorbed it, and remembered it? Somehow, you made a decision to remember it because you had an important reason for doing so, whether you wanted to excel at your job or you had an important test to pass. Whatever the reason, your learning increased because you had the motivation or a purpose for learning it.

Motivation to learn is a key ingredient in presetting your mind for learning. If you take a few seconds at the start of any learning session and say, "What is my purpose or goal for learning this material?" you will have programmed your mind to be attentive and interested. The more relevant the subject is to your life, the greater the chance you have for keeping your attention fully on the subject.

Determine why you need to learn the subject you selected and keep this goal in mind as you learn the new material.

Exercise: Write down your reason for learning the subject.

What Do I Already Know About the Subject?
___

The next step in the planning stage of your learning is to evaluate what you already know about the subject. To accelerate your learning you will need to fit the instruction into the shortest possible time. One way to do that is to eliminate wasting time relearning what you already know. Time and life are too short to sit through the same material repeatedly. You want to focus on new information.

To make this evaluation, list what you already know about the subject. Only write down what you are sure that you know because you may need a refresher for some material. As you go through your learning program, you can skip or skim over what you already know to save time.

Exercise: Write down what you already know about the subject:

What Do I Need to Know About This Subject?
___

After determining what you already know, the next step is to evaluate what you *need* to know about the subject. Most people go blindly into a subject. They plod along from one point to the next, starting at the front cover of a book and ending at the back. If the book contains topics not relevant, you should skip them to avoid being slowed down.

If you are taking a course, an instructor can guide you as to what you need to learn. If you are doing a self-study program, you need to do some preparation in advance and find out what you want to know about the subject. Do you want to master a certain process or skill and cover certain topics? Do you want to show proficiency in one area or know everything that was ever written about that subject? Decide what it is you need to know to satisfy your goals. List those topics and use that list as your guide. In this way, you can select the most helpful material and skip what is irrelevant to your learning plan.

Exercise: Write down what you need to know about the subject.

Exercise: Review the information on your kinesthetic Superlink learning style and brain style described in this book and list the best learning methods and materials for you to learn.

How Can I Use Positive Thinking to Learn Anything Quickly and Raise My Confidence and Self-esteem?

If you had a hard time learning in school, you may not have enough confidence in yourself and your abilities. Perhaps you saw others earn high grades while you received low grades or even failed. This may have resulted in low self-esteem, negative thoughts about yourself, or thinking there is something wrong with you. Unfortunately, years of this kind of negative attitude may become a self-fulfilling prophecy. When we think we can't do something, we put so much energy into that negative thought that we may end up not succeeding. On the other hand, when we think we can succeed, we work with confidence and end up succeeding.

One study conducted by Harvard researchers, led by Robert Rosenthal, and that later became known as "Pygmalion in the Classroom," focused on a group of ninety students of average ability. Three teachers to whom they were assigned in classes of thirty each were told that they were gifted students. The teachers, thinking that they had gifted students, taught them as if they *were* gifted and had high expectations of them. At the end of the study, the progress of each group was measured. The results were that the students met those expectations, did exceedingly well, and their achievement soared. (Canter, Lee, and Canter, Marlene. *The High Performing Teacher; Avoiding Burnout and Increasing Your Motivation*: A Publication of Lee Canter and Associates, Santa

Monica, CA. 1994, pp. 25-26). What this study points out is that our performance can be influenced by our expectations of ourselves as well as others' expectations of us.

You might have been slowed down because you were not taught in your kinesthetic Superlinks learning style and brain style. You learned quickly in the first few years of life because you were allowed to use your natural way of learning—the learning method that is easiest for you—which may have been any of the following: exploring, playing, learning games, hands-on learning, or any other method. But in traditional schools, students must learn in one or two ways, mostly by watching (a visual method) or listening to the teacher (an auditory one). If students do not have the same learning style as the one used in the classroom they struggle to learn. During the time they spend trying to adapt to a learning style that is not compatible with their own, the class has already moved on. These students do not know what is wrong with them or why others are getting it and they are not. They do not know that if they were taught in a learning style and brain style that matched their own they would move along as quickly as some of the other students. But the students do not know what to ask for. They are prisoners of a system that is not working for them.

If you are one of those who experienced failure or felt you could not learn as quickly as others, or were a good student and wanted to be better and could not, you were probably just as bright as those other children, but were limited by a learning method that was not compatible with your own. The students who did well may have been those whose Superlink matched the teacher's presentation. If you were to take those who did well and put them in a learning environment that is not compatible with their learning style, they also might struggle or find it harder to achieve.

How can we raise our self-esteem? First, realize that *every* human being has an amazing capacity to learn. In the first seven years of life, children can learn an entire language and the meaning of thousands of words. Our brain does not shut down after first grade. There is nothing inherent in any of us that says that we suddenly become incapable of learning when we arrive at the doors of an elementary school. The same brain that you used to assimilate an entire language in the first seven years of life is just as intelligent and prepared to learn after it begins school. To raise your self-esteem, realize that what happened to you in the past may not have been your fault. Had you been taught in your kinesthetic learning style and brain style you would have learned faster and more easily. What is past is past and now you know how *you* need to learn. Start from today. Feel confident that you now have an approach that will work for you. As you begin to learn through the approach that matches your Superlink learning style and brain style, you will experience the feeling that others who have done so have also experienced—you *can* do it. It is easy, fun, and natural. Having positive learning experiences will help you to start feeling good about yourself. Slowly, those feelings of past failures will fade.

You need to start a cycle of success. How is this done? Firstly, think of a time in which you succeeded at a task. It could have been a school subject, an extracurricular activity, or something you did on your own at home. Try to relive the experience in your mind. How did it feel to succeed? Did you feel happy, proud, and confident? Did you want to repeat the experience? Most people would say they would like to repeat the task because of the good feelings that accompanied the experience.

Now think of a time when you failed at something. It could have been a school subject, a sport or hobby, or something you did at home. How did you feel? Did you feel hurt, angry, frustrated, stupid, or hopeless? Did you want to repeat that task again? Most people, unless they wanted to repeat it just to prove to themselves they could do it, would say they did not want to repeat the task. Thus, because of the pain of the experience, they began to avoid the very area in which they may have needed to practice. The more they avoided practicing, the further they grew from mastering it. The cycle of failure began. The initial failure caused them to avoid the task, get further behind, and reinforced more failure.

It is time to break the cycle. By learning according to your kinesthetic Superlink learning style and brain style, you will now find it easier to learn. Gain confidence. Start with some easy work to regain the good feelings that come with success. Then, as you find you can finally succeed, slowly add harder and more challenging material. Do not frustrate yourself by beginning with material that is too hard. Until you regain your self-esteem, master the technique of learning in your best Superlink learning style using some review material. Then add new material as you regain confidence.

Whatever your level of education, know that you carry in your head a most remarkable computer. You just have to fit compatible software into the hardware of your brain for it to run properly. Many others who have tried these methods have succeeded, and you can, too!

Exercise: Tell yourself, "I can raise my self-esteem and positive thoughts about myself by realizing the possible causes of my previous struggles with learning." List subjects with which you previously had trouble, analyze how they were taught and how the methods may not have been compatible with your kinesthetic learning style. List methods from this book compatible with your kinesthetic Superlink learning style and brain style that could have been used to make those subjects easier to learn.

Why Are Relaxation and Stress Reduction Techniques Important?

Relaxation and stress reduction can accelerate learning. Medical research over the past decades has been exploring the connection between the mind and body. When we are in a state of fear or extreme stress, the body's survival reaction is to shut down our higher-level thinking portion and respond according to the part of the brain that deals with the fight or flight response. We respond with physiological reactions such as increases of adrenaline, rapid heartbeats, and constricted blood vessels. Your body is readying itself to run or fight, requiring the use of your arms and legs. During this state, you are not ready to remember a mathematical theorem or new vocabulary words.

People who had negative experiences of failure in the classroom enter into this state of panic and fear when it comes to learning. Test taking may cause them to be fearful so they do not score well even if they studied. Their teachers or parents may have been upset with them, inflicted physical, psychological, or emotional pain and punishment, called them demeaning names, or ostracized them because of their mistakes at school. Years of reliving this trauma may cause people to enter a state of stress, panic, and fear when they have to learn something new. For successful learning to take place we need to learn how to relax and reduce stress. We have to program ourselves to break the cycle of failure and get out of the habit of fearing learning. Relaxation and stress-reduction techniques can assist in the process.

Step one is to put the past behind you, realize that these struggles with learning or test taking may not have been entirely your fault, and remind yourself that the fear response is only a habit. You now know what you need in order to learn; things *will* be different this time. By following a new approach that suits your style, you will be more successful. So relax—this time you *will* succeed!

Step two is to get your body into a physiological state of relaxation. Our brain waves run at different frequencies. From thirteen to twenty Hz (Hertz) or cps (cycles per second) we are in the beta state, the state in which we function at work, driving, or in the fight-or-flight mode. From nine to twelve Hz we are in the alpha state, in which we are more relaxed, but alert. The alpha state is good for learning. The theta state, from five to eight Hz, is the meditation state. That is good for relaxation and stress reduction. From one to four Hz we are in the delta state, which is deep sleep. Before learning, we may want to reduce our stress and increase our relaxation by entering into the theta state—the state of meditation. There are different ways to do this.

One way to reach the state of relaxation is to slow down our breathing. In fear, the hormones we release increase our heart rate. To reduce a rapid heart rate and to relax, find a place to sit in a relaxed position. Take some deep breaths, letting the air fill your lungs. Breathe to the count of four, hold for four, and release your breath in four. Do this slow breathing for several minutes, until you feel your heartbeat slow down. As you breathe in, feel relaxation enter you, filling your entire body. Imagine being filled with this relaxation. Feel your stress evaporate as calm and peace fill you. Imagine that relaxation opens you up to receive the wisdom and knowledge to help you learn anything you want to know. You can then feel the stress of your body disappear and relaxation fill you.

Another way to get to the theta state is to still your mind and eliminate all thoughts of panic, worry, and fear. Sitting for a few minutes in meditation calms your mind. Close your eyes and sit in a relaxed manner. Do not think about anything; just concentrate within. A feeling of relaxation will come over your body and mind. By keeping your attention within, you will find your powers of concentration become focused and sharp. You may feel a sense of peace. Some people even experience blissful joy. Your worries and fears melt away—you are now in the state where you are ready to learn.

Some people try a variety of other techniques for relaxation. Some use music to get into this state. Early work with accelerated learning developed by the Bulgarian researcher Georgi Lozanov relied on music to get the mind ready for learning. Baroque music, which contains sixty beats per minute, supposedly synchronizes with the heartbeat, helping people get into an optimal learning state. Musician Steven Halpern has found that music with less than sixty beats per minute also works. His research reveals that music with a slower beat slows the heart rate, putting the body and mind into a more relaxed state, ideal for learning. He has been a pioneer in producing music to accelerate learning. Some schools have used his music to create a calm, peaceful state in which students can learn with a stress-free attitude.

Some people like to do physical exercise or yoga to get the

body relaxed. Exercise or physical yoga stimulates the flow of oxygen through the bloodstream, carrying it to the brain to eliminate mental stress and get the brain ready for learning. New research reveals that exercise stimulates the brain to make more connections that can increase learning and improve memory.

Whatever method you use, the end result is to calm the body and mind to keep them out of the fight-or-flight mode. Before beginning a learning session, spend five or ten minutes in any of the relaxation techniques. You can do the same one every day, or you can vary them. Find those that work the best for you. The goal is to keep the higher-thinking functions in the brain open so that learning can take place.

Exercise: Try different stress-reduction activities to find those that are best for you.

How Can I Visualize Success?

The last step in the planning stage for learning is to visualize success. New studies have shown that even thinking about doing a task results in neuron connections being made as if they had physically performed the activity. This is a powerful discovery supported by scientific evidence indicating that by mentally going through a task, brain cells are forming connections for that task, accelerating our learning and improving our memory. Athletes have been using this technique for years. Before a competition, they visualize or imagine themselves winning. The power of a positive mental mind-set and pre-setting brain connections for success is used in other fields as well. Medical researchers and doctors have reported cases in which after the visualization of good health, their patients' health improved. Health and wellness centers around the world have been established, devoted to helping people visualize themselves becoming healthy. The same technique has been used for increasing learning, reading and listening comprehension, and memory.

The technique is simple. Sit quietly in a relaxed state. You can get into a meditative state first so that the body and mind are calm and stilled. Select the following next steps as a kinesthetic learner.

The kinesthetic learner will experience themselves jumping up and giving a victory punch with their fist into the air and saying, "Yes!" after successfully completing the course. Try to make the image of your successful moment as vivid as possible, using all your senses, with your kinesthetic Superlink learning style and brain style as the main modality. Imagine yourself being actively engaged in some action as a result of your successful learning. Live the successful moment as if it really has already happened. Repeat this activity daily. Know that you have already succeeded. Live each day as one more step leading to the success that is already yours. Students have successfully used this technique to win scholarships or admission into schools in which the competition was fierce.

Visualizing your success as well as doing the steps in this accelerated program of how to learn anything quickly to improve kinesthetic memory go hand in hand. The visualization of success adds the power of positive thinking to the tools you are learning. You are now ready to learn quickly the subject you have chosen to master.

Exercise: Visualize yourself succeeding at quickly learning the subject you chose and write a description of what you visualized yourself doing kinesthetically.

CHAPTER 5:
CHOOSING A KINESTHETIC LEARNER'S BEST INSTRUCTION, MATERIALS, AND LEARNING ENVIRONMENT TO IMPROVE MEMORY TO LEARN ANYTHING QUICKLY

After preparing your mind for optimum learning, you are ready to begin taking in the information you need to learn quickly to improve memory. You will discover:

- how instruction should be delivered to fit your kinesthetic Superlink learning style and brain style.
- the learning materials you should use for your unique kinesthetic Superlink.
- the learning environment you need for your kinesthetic Superlink learning style.
- how to convert information from your weaker Superlink learning style to your kinesthetic style.

You want to choose the type of instruction, learning materials, and learning environment that will allow you to absorb information that matches your kinesthetic Superlink learning style in order to learn quickly.

If you have control over your learning plan, you can make the above decisions about the type of information yourself. In many cases, though, you will be learning from others, such as through a course, a required manual, or a curriculum prescribed for your training in your field of work. Some of the above decisions may not rest in your hands but are left up to the instructor or the institution preparing your learning program. The people teaching you may not do so in a way that matches your kinesthetic learning style and brain style. In that case, you have two options. The first option is to explain to the instructor or coordinator of your studies how you learn best and ask him or her to present the material in a way that is compatible with your kinesthetic Superlink learning and brain style. The second option comes into play when the instructor or coordinator does not want to or cannot present the material in your kinesthetic style. In that case, you need to learn how to convert the type of instruction to your kinesthetic learning style and brain style. This chapter will teach you how to do this. This ability can be a powerful tool that will enable you to in *any* situation—you won't need to rely on others to determine whether or not you succeed.

Fit the Instruction and Materials to Your Kinesthetic Superlink Learning Style and Brain Style

There are many ways to learn a subject. The medium of instruction and the materials are the communication methods used to convey the material. Below are some of the different instructional media and materials.

Written material: books, eBooks, digital downloads, PDFs, textbooks, manuals, guidebooks, booklets, pamphlets, reference materials such as encyclopedias, almanacs, dictionaries, thesauruses, magazines, journals, newspaper, microfilm, microfiche, scripts, screenplays, poetry, charts, lists, diagrams, graphs, faxed material, emails, blogs, ezine articles, Internet postings, websites, etc.

Graphic material: photographs, illustrations, pictures, drawings, maps, atlases, posters, cartoons, diagrams and charts with graphics, digital graphic downloads, graphic ebooks, PDFs, websites with graphics, illustrated aps, etc.

Audio-Visual Material: apps, digital audio downloads, streaming audio over the Internet, audiotapes, CDs, slides, power-point, filmstrips, DVDs, streaming videos, 3-D movies, radio, television, distance learning through teleconferencing, web conferences, web meetings, and webinars, cable television, educational television, and public broadcasting.

From Computers: information from the Internet, streaming video and audio, software programs, apps, virtual reality, webinars, web conferences, telesemimars, social media, e-mail, distance learning via computer, and on-line courses and degrees programs.

Hands-on Activities: writing, typing, drawing, sketching, painting, creating graphics on the computer, sculpture, building, constructing, arts and crafts, using tools, machinery or equipment, role-playing, simulations, learning games, using manipulatives, dramatization, film-making, video production, theater productions, music productions, demonstrations, making discoveries, exploration, performing experiments, sports, exercises, etc.

Real-life Experiences: on-the-job training, fieldwork, trips to museums, learning centers (such as oceanariums, seaquariums, forest preserves, or environmental centers), or engaging in apprenticeships in stores or retail businesses, service industries, construction sites, hospitals, schools, factories, farms, delivery companies, airports, shipyards, railway stations, banks, the stock exchange, supermarkets, auto repair shops, art studios, theater or dance companies, concert halls, etc.), playing on sports teams (football, baseball, basketball, soccer, hockey, golf, etc.), or engaging in training programs coordinated between places of employment and schools, etc.

Personal Instructors: direct instruction from teachers, professors, instructors, guides, mentors, life coaches, athletic or sports coaches, certified personal trainers, facilitators, trainers, skilled craftspeople, employers, managers or supervisors. (The person may instruct through oral presentations or lectures, reading aloud material to the students or requiring students to read it themselves, providing printed graphic material, audio-visual material, and computer technology, setting up hands-on learning activities, or putting the learners into real-life situations in order to learn.)

Combinations of the above: Any of the above teaching methods can be combined.

Based on the description of your Superlink that you read in this book, choose the instructional medium and materials from the above lists that corresponds with your kinesthetic Superlink learning style and brain style.

If you can control your learning, then you can set it up in the way that will help you learn quickly. But we do not always have control over the way we are instructed. We may not be in charge of choosing the best medium or learning material, or selecting the learning environment. Is it hopeless? Absolutely not. What you can do is convert any instruction into your own best kinesthetic Superlink learning style. You can still learn even if the medium, material, and environment do not suit your style. The following pages show you the instructional media compatible with your kinesthetic learning style and how to convert medium not in your style into your kinesthetic Superlink. Think of it as a translation system to show you what you can do to turn a poor situation into an optimal one.

The following information will enable you to convert a

medium of instruction and materials or some aspect of them into the best medium of instruction and materials for a kinesthetic Superlink.

Converting Instruction and Materials into Kinesthetic Learning Style and Brain Style to Improve Memory

Superlink: Kinesthetic Left Brain Learners:
Media Type:
Written Material: Have the learner act out the words in a step-by-step way or imagine the action in their mind, feeling it in their muscles.

Graphic Material: Have the learner physically act out the graphic representation or imagine the action in their mind in a step-by-step way, while feeling it in their muscles.

Audio-Visual Material: Have the learner dramatize or imagine acting out what they see and hear as an action in their mind, feeling it in their muscles, in a step-by-step way.

Computers: Have the learner physically act out the written text or graphics shown on the computer, or imagine doing the action, while feeling it in their muscles, in a step-by-step way.

Hands-On Activities: Hands-on activities need to also be carried out physically, or have the learner imagine doing the action in their mind, feeling it in their muscles, in a step-by-step way.

Real-Life Experiences: Ideal for kinesthetic left brain learners. Use as a step-by-step approach and put it into words.

Learning from an Instructor: For visual, auditory, or tactile presentations, the learner can carry them out physically or imagine the action in their mind, feeling it in their muscles, in a step-by-step way, putting in into words.

Superlink: Kinesthetic Right Brain Learners:
Media Type:

Written Material: Have the learner physically act out the words or imagine doing the action in their mind, feeling it in their muscles.

Graphic Material: Have the learner physically act out the graphic representation or imagine doing the action in their mind, feeling it in their muscles.

Audio-Visual Material: Carry out the actions physically that they see and hear or imagine the action in their mind, while feeling it in their muscles.

Computers: Written text or graphics need to be physically carried out, or have the learner imagine the action in their mind, feeling it in their muscles, with freedom of movement and imagination.

Hands-On Activities: For visual, auditory, and tactile activities, have the learner participate in the experience physically or imagine doing the action, feeling it in their muscles, with freedom of movement and imagination.

Real-Life Experiences: This is ideal for kinesthetic right brain learners. Use a global approach, beginning with the big picture, main idea, or overview.

Learning from an Instructor: For visual, auditory, or tactile instruction, have the learner physically act it out or imagine doing the action in their mind, while feeling it in their muscles, with freedom of movement and imagination.

In summary, each type of instruction and learning material can be made suitable for any type of learner. There is no reason for books and graphic materials to be made only for visual people; books can be produced to appeal to auditory, tactile, and kinesthetic people who are either left brain or right brain or both. As a consultant and a writer of learning materials for many years, I have developed programs that deliver instruction through the medium that matches the learners' best Superlink learning style and brain style. For example, I created an entire pre-K, K-12, college and adult reading program, called Keys to Reading Success and Superlinks to Accelerated Learning with lessons in all eight Superlinks styles so everyone can excel in reading, reading and listening comprehension, vocabulary, phonics, fluency, memory, note taking, study skills, and test-taking skills. Any medium can be converted to match the learner's style.

Exercise: Review the chapter on your kinesthetic Superlink and then use the above information to find your best media of instruction and materials that matches your kinesthetic Superlink learning style. Take notes of all the instructional methods and media materials that match your kinesthetic learning style and brain style to improve memory.

The Learning Environment You Need

Your learning environment refers to where you will work, read, or study: the conditions in the room and other stimuli that can enhance or inhibit your ability to learn. You may have set yourself up with the right delivery of instruction and the right materials, but if your environment causes you discomfort or distractions it will be harder to concentrate. To improve memory to accelerate learning you want to eliminate as many steps that block your progress as possible.

When you set up your own environment, you can control

your circumstances. But when you are in a training or class situation, you may not have control over your environment. Thus, you may have to ask the instructor for some assistance in making some adjustments in the environment, or use coping techniques to help you adapt to the situation.

Below is a list summarizing the best learning environment to improve memory for the kinesthetic left brain or right brain learner followed by coping skills for adapting a noncompatible environment into one that is compatible for you.

Superlink: Kinesthetic Left Brain Learners:
Best Learning Environment:
- Plenty of space to stretch out and move around.
- Freedom to get out of their seat or work standing up.
- Comfortable seats.
- White boards or flip charts allow them to stand up and write.
- Neat, organized surroundings.
- Time schedules.

Coping Strategies to Adapt a Noncompatible Environment:
- Sit near the back of the room so they can move around without distracting anyone.
- If they have to sit to work, use a chair in which they can lean back, stretch out, wiggle, or move a lot.
- Ask for a time schedule. Wear a watch.

- Bring a challenging game or activity or something to do quietly at their seat if they get bored after finishing work earlier than others and have to wait for the next part of the lesson.
- If they like music, bring headphones so as not to disturb others.
- Do arm or leg exercises at their seat if they get bored or restless.
- When studying, stay in a study carrel or put up a book or divider to block out the distraction of others' movements, or face a wall.

Superlink: Kinesthetic Right Brain Learners:
Best Learning Environment:
- Enough space to move around and stretch out.
- Freedom to get out of their seat or work standing up.
- Comfortable places with room to stretch out on the floor or couch, and if sitting is required, use chairs on which they can lean back, stretch their legs, wiggle, or move.
- Places to play learning or movement games.
- Permission to work with or without music.
- When studying, sit at a study carrel or have a divider to block out the view of others' movements and activities.
- White boards, flip charts, or smart boards allow them to stand up and write.

- Flexible time schedule, and if work is done, allowed to leave early or keep working, if they want, well past the finishing time.
- Competitions, rewards, and awards for achieving a goal.

Coping Strategies to Adapt to a Noncompatible Environment:
- Select a place where they can move around without disturbing others, preferable at the back of the room.
- Make sure if they have to sit, the seat allows for leaning back, stretching their legs, wiggling, and moving around.
- Bring a challenging game or activity, or something to do quietly when bored while waiting for the next task if they finish before others in a class or training.
- If they like music while learning, provide headphones so as not to disturb others.
- Work at a study carrel or use a book or divider to block out distractions from others' movements or actions.
- Keep a color-coded calendar or use sticky-notes as reminders of time schedules.

Exercise: Use some of the above suggestions for your kinesthetic Superlink learning style and brain style and apply them to learning any subject quickly.

Chapter 6:

Strategies to Improve a Kinesthetic Learner's Memory

Training Your Memory

We have a tremendous amount of data stored in our brain that we can pull up at will. One reason we do not remember certain things is that we did not make an *effort* to remember them longer for an extended period of time. Consciously or unconsciously, we *chose* to remember those items we do remember. If we want to improve our memory, we can do so by training ourselves to remember what we want when we want.

When we talk of learning anything quickly, we want to learn the subject as well as recall it for more than just a moment. Sadly, when many instructors teach a subject, the students know it only until they are tested on it. Give them a surprise test a month or two later and all that hard work to learn the subject seems to have been for naught. How is it possible that we can spend six months to a year taking a course and forget what we learned years later? It is not that we do not have a good memory—we just do not have a *trained* memory. Accelerated learning involves training our memory using our Superlink learning style and brain style.

Long-term and Short-term Memory

We have two memory systems: short-term and long-term memory.

Short-term memory holds something temporarily in our mind until we decide what to do with it. Consciously or unconsciously, we can either decide to store it in our long-term memory or dismiss it as something unimportant. Our short-term memory is a revolving door with new information entering continually. It can be compared to a computer screen memory. Information stays there as long as we are focusing on it and working with it. Then we must decide whether to save it in the hard drive—the computer's long-term memory—or let it be erased when we turn the computer off.

Long-term memory permanently holds something in our memory. There are many things we learned in childhood that were placed in our long-term memory that we have not forgotten: walking; riding a bicycle, speaking our language, writing the alphabet, or singing childhood songs and nursery rhymes, among other things. These memories become a part of our database from which we can draw at any time.

Keys to Improving Your Kinesthetic Memory

The basics of having a good memory are simple and can be learned by people of any age, including young children. You *can* improve your kinesthetic memory.

Step 1) Having a purpose or goal for remembering what you are learning.

Step 2) Consciously deciding to put what you learn into long-term memory.

Step 3) Use your kinesthetic Superlink learning style and brain style to store what you learn in your long-term memory.

Step 4) Keeping your memory active by retrieving it and using it.

Step 1: Having a Purpose or Goal for Remembering What You Are Learning

We are bombarded with millions of bits of information daily. With the advent of the Internet, the information superhighway, we have access to a huge amount of information circulating through the world on a daily basis. If we were to recall every single sensory impression and bit of information we receive we would be so overwhelmed we would not be able to focus on the range of activities that were more important to our lives. Life is too short to learn everything about everything; we must make a conscious choice about what we want to remember. This process involves deciding why we need to learn something. When we want to learn something, we must also decide why it is important for us to learn it. If we keep that goal in mind, we will put our brain on notice that this is material we *want* to remember.

Why did you remember your name as a child? When you figured out that people kept asking you your name, you decided that next time they asked you had better know it or they may think there is something wrong with you. Why did you learn those twenty-six meaningless sounds called the "alphabet" when you were just a toddler? You had no idea what they stood for or what words they went with, but you learned how to repeat these twenty-six sounds that might well have been nonsense to you. Why did you learn it? Maybe you figured out that your parents would show you off to their friends by having you repeat the alphabet and would give you that big smile and hug that you loved. Or maybe you surmised that your relatives would give you a monetary award for being such a "good and smart" child for saying your "ABCs." You had a purpose for learning that information at age two, three, or four, which had nothing to do with getting a high school diploma. You could have just as easily been taught the ABCs in a foreign language, or the periodic table of the elements, or the names of all the bones of the body. We learned what we did because someone valued it, rewarded us for knowing it with either verbal or nonverbal gestures or material gifts, and this made us feel good.

The same principle holds true today when it comes to learning. You really wanted to learn how to drive so you mastered the physical act of driving, while remembering the driver's manual with all its facts, figures, and state laws. The same people who cannot pass a social studies test can pass a written driving examination on technical information and legal terms. Why? They wanted to remember the driver's education manual because it meant if they could learn how to drive they could have wheels. It is the same brain that is reading that driver's education manual that is reading other textbooks. Is there a selective gene in our body that discriminates between learning a driver's education manual and a political science course? Not at all. It is our intention and desire to learn something that determines what we will remember and what we will forget.

Some possible reasons, purposes, or goals for learning are: to get a job or advance in our career; to improve our skills; to raise our salary; to get a promotion; to become certified in a field; to pass a test; to keep up with new knowledge; to help others; for enjoyment, personal growth or curiosity; or for many other reasons.

Exercise: Take the subject you chose to study as you worked through this book and write a sentence or two stating why you want to learn more about this subject.

Step 2: Consciously Decide to Put What You Learn into Your Long-Term Kinesthetic Memory

We must program our minds to send information into our long-term kinesthetic memory if we wish to retain it. Otherwise, we will get the information, comprehend it, but it will be erased shortly afterwards. If we want to recall it for the long haul, we have to establish the reason for wanting to put it into long-term kinesthetic memory and the length of time we want it to stay in memory. Many people find they lack study skills and test-taking skills because they cannot remember what they read, hear, or study long enough to pass a test. That is because they do not program themselves to recall everything they learn for the entire duration of the course of study.

Here are some things to think about when you are trying to commit what you want learn to your long-term kinesthetic memory:

1) If you learn it the first time you read or hear it you won't have to go over the material again and again, wasting precious time.

2) You can use what you learn to work towards your job promotion, advancement, or passing a test, certification exam, or course faster.

3) You will have more free time to do other things.

4) You will be able to use the information right away.

Decide that you want to commit what you learn to your long-term kinesthetic memory, the length of time you want to retain it, and why it is important for you to learn it.

Exercise: Using the subject you selected to learn as you work through this book, write your reasons for putting what you learn about the subject into long-term memory.

Step 3: Use Your Superlink Learning Style and Brain Style to Store What You Learn in Your Long-Term Memory

This is the key to the entire process. I developed this technique as an extension of the application of Superlinks learning styles and brain styles. It works so incredibly quickly that everyone who has used it is amazed at how sharp his or her memory becomes.

The secret is: The key to improving your memory and remembering what you learn is to store it according to your kinesthetic Superlink learning style and brain style.

Kinesthetic learners remember best what you did and how your body moved. **Kinesthetic people** would *act out* the actions and events of the movie in their minds.

By experiencing what you read or hear using your kinesthetic Superlink learning style and brain style, you are causing your mind to think an event is really happening to you. You have involved yourself into a true virtual reality experience that is taking place inside your mind through your best sense, supported by the other senses.

Books or lectures are real events that have been converted into words for the benefit of those who were not there. Writing is like creating a cyberworld in which reality is encoded into words, and reading decodes or converts it back into experiences and events. Reading is like cracking a code so we can recreate the writer or speaker's experience in our minds. The more vividly we do this and the more we involve ourselves in the action, the more we will experience being there and the more thoroughly we will remember it.

There is a passage you can use for reading comprehension and memory practice is given below in Exercise 1. As you read, make a commitment to put this information into long-term memory. Attempt to remember *all* the details of this passage, including names, dates, and other factual information. Read it according to your kinesthetic Superlink learning style and brain style. Convert it into a movie in your mind feeling it. Make associations for words, numbers, and dates, finding similar words or images already in your mind.

After reading the passage, cover it up and discover how much of it you remember now that you have experienced it as an actual event. If you imagined the story in your kinesthetic Superlink learning style and brain style, you should have found that you can answer every question and recall every detail after converting it into a movie scene based on your preferred sense. If you missed any questions or details, analyze why. Most likely you did not make a strong enough experience in your mind or you skipped over part of the text without imagining it. It is always fascinating to find that any text that a kinesthetic learner did not imagine as a movie in their best kinesthetic Superlink learning style is gone from his or her memory when he or she tries to answer the questions, while the material that the person *did* imagine in his or her kinesthetic Superlink style pops out as if he or she really experienced the event.

You can do this kind of reading with everything you read, fiction or nonfiction, including informational texts. You can try this with reading the daily news whether printed in a newspaper or Internet news site, magazine or ezine articles, trade journals, memos, newsletters, interoffice communications, text messages, email, faxes, flogs, social media sites, or websites. The same technique can work with a novel as well as with scientific material, technical reading, history, the social sciences, health, medical books, training materials for any field, textbooks on any subjects, or anything else you can think of. You can also use it for listening comprehension when listening to lectures. Auditory left brain people are good at mentally recording material directly in their minds, but those with a kinesthetic Superlinks learning style and brain style would take dictation only for the purpose of converting the material into an experiential event later at their own pace in their own quickest way of learning.

Anyone can train themselves to read or listen to any material and put it into long-term memory. What does it take? All you have to do is be mentally present as you read. The moment you just look at the words without converting them, you have actually stopped reading. Reading only takes place when the words become images or experiences in your mind. Unless you are an auditory left brain person who gets meaning directly from words, without converting them into corresponding experiences in your kinesthetic Superlink learning style and brain style, just reading (for a kinesthetic learning style) "word, word, word, word" continually without imagining kinesthetic movement is not only NOT READING, it may be a boring, useless task that does not help you because you are not comprehending. Begin to monitor your reading by making sure you are converting every word you read into kinesthetic experiences in your mind. Remember, the moment you stop making movie scenes in your kinesthetic Superlink learning style and brain style, you have stopped reading. You have begun to daydream or mentally wander. Every word you may have looked at or even said aloud while your mind wandered and did not imagine kinesthetic movement is gone from your memory because you were not really mentally present. You will then need to return to the last set of words that you imaged and reread that section using the virtual reality experiential kinesthetic reading comprehension technique or it may be lost.

If you are reading to learn, you will soon realize that when you do not mentally act out the text as you read, you are wasting precious time. Not only do you *not* comprehend the information, you will not be sending it into long-term kinesthetic memory. That is why you may have had to read the same material over and over in the past. But if you are in a hurry and want to learn anything quickly, you need to read it correctly the first time around. You will find that with a little practice you can have total recall and memory of everything you read. Just be attentive, do the conversion process in your kinesthetic learning style and brain style, and with hardly any effort, the whole passage will come back to you hours, days, or even weeks later because you transformed it into an experience that happened to you. This method of kinesthetic reading comprehension and memory that I developed and tested with people of all ages is a powerful tool you will have to speed up your reading and learning.

As you answered the reading comprehension questions for the sample passage, you may have noticed that as certain key words in the questions came up, a movement memory arose in your mind. If you are not auditory and you tried to remember the words, you may have drawn a blank. But if you instead said to yourself, "What did I experience or feel my muscles doing in my movie?" while you were in a relaxed mental state, the movie would have rerun in your head and the answer would have appeared. You were using both your right and left hemisphere of the brain in this process. The movement or action appears in the side of the brain that can picture yourself doing it (usually the right side of the brain), and the word or words describing yourself doing it is recalled from your speech and language centers in the brain (usually the left side of the brain, although some people have some language in the right side of the brain). This combined in the kinesthetic part of your brain that recalls movement. Thus, you have engaged your whole brain in this process. This kind of kinesthetic reading comprehension and memory is a great exercise for developing your whole brain. You are making more connections between the two halves of the brain and developing your thinking and memory powers as well.

Memory Improvement

Exercise 1: You can use this sample passage to practice the experiential virtual reality reading comprehension and memory technique in your kinesthetic Superlinks learning style and brain style, or, if you grasp how it works, you can move on to Exercise 2 to practice it with an actual subject you want to read or study.

Next, I will model for you how we can work together through the following sample practice kinesthetic reading comprehension and memory passage, "Dave," making a commitment in our minds that we want to put this information into long-term memory. The task is to attempt to remember *all* the details of this passage, including names, dates, and other factual details. We are going to read it according to your kinesthetic Superlink learning style and brain style. I am going to involve both sides of your brain, the right and left side, for this exercise to show you how you can remember both the big picture and graphic images (right brain functions) as well as every detail and the words for the experience (left brain functions). Thus, we are going to engage both sides of the brain in the process of reading the sample passage called "Dave." Although the entire passage appears below, do not read it yet, but skip down to "Instructions for Reading the Sample Practice Kinesthetic Reading Comprehension and Memory Passage: 'Dave'" and let it guide you to read the sample passage in small chunks as directed.

Note: For those who teach, coach, or mentor others, please see my other books in this series that focus on how to model teaching this Virtual Reality Comprehension and Memory passage to tactile, visual, and auditory learners. (See *How to Quickly Improve Memory and Learning for Tactile Left and Right Brain Superlinks Learning Styles; How to Quickly Improve Memory and Learning for Visual Left and Right Brain Superlinks Learning Styles;* and *How to Quickly Improve Memory and Learning for Auditory Left and Right Brain Superlinks Learning Styles.* If you want an edition that contains all the different learning and brain styles memory techniques combined in one volume, you can go to *How to Improve Memory Quickly through the Brain's Fastest Superlinks Learning Styles.* The individual learning style editions were requested by those who just wanted to focus on their own or one style.)

Sample Practice Kinesthetic Reading Comprehension and Memory Passage: "Dave"

Dave looked at his watch as he rushed out of his apartment. It was Monday morning and he was late again. As he ran down the steps of his apartment building, heading towards his red sports car, he felt the humid air pressing in on him. It was going to be another hot summer day in June. Dave opened his car door, tossed his brown attaché case onto the passenger seat, and slid into the driver's side. This was the only thing he looked forward to every morning, driving his new car along the freeway to his office. He looked forward to next week when he would begin a two-week vacation. As he drove towards Interstate 72, his mind raced along thinking about his holiday. "Aruba sounds good with its dry air, its seventy-degree weather, and its cool ocean breezes—a change from this stifling humidity," he thought to himself. A short ring from his cell phone startled him out of his daydream.

Kinesthetic Instructions for Reading the Sample Passage "Dave": Now, we are going to read through this passage together, using your kinesthetic Superlink learning style and brain style to convert this into an experience that you will save in your long-term memory. As we read, visual people will *see* what is happening, auditory people will *hear* what is happening, tactile people will *feel* what is happening, but kinesthetic people will be experiencing *doing* the actions of what is happening. Ready to roll the scene? You can make it a movie, a theater production, or a real-life event happening to you. Ready? Lights, camera, action:

The passage first says: "Dave looked at his watch as he rushed out of his apartment." Make an image in your mind of Dave. Think of someone named Dave that you know, either a personal relationship or an actor, athlete, or someone famous, so you can remember his name and put that person into the movie. Next pretend to act out being Dave by becoming the Dave you pictured for this movie and act out the scenes in your mind. When the passage mentions the watch, imagine yourself as Dave doing an action with a watch. Describe an action you would do with a watch in your kinesthetic Superlink learning style (for example, kinesthetic learners may experience themselves taking off the watch, propping it up on a table, and doing a physical exercise in time to the movement of the secondhand of the watch). Next, experience yourself rushing out of your apartment. Based on your kinesthetic Superlink learning style, you may imagine an action you would do; for example, swinging open the door and racing down the steps.

Read the next phrase: "It was Monday morning...." Think, "How will you remember Monday morning? What actions come to you when you think of Monday? How would you portray Monday in the form of an action on a movie screen to let the audience know that it is Monday?" Kinesthetic learners may feel their car speed up and slow down in the stop and go traffic as they drive to work during Monday morning rush-hour traffic. Alternatively, they may think of how that on Monday night they would be watching their favorite football team play on "Monday Night Football." The key is to think of an association that will help them remember the word "Monday."

Now read the next phrase: "...and he was late again." Create an action associated with being "late again." For example, imagine being late because you stopped to throw a few basketballs in a hoop or jogging with a friend before work. Now, experience rushing home to change clothes to dress for work with the clock's hand moving past the time you should have already left for work to be on time. Feel your muscles tightening up in preparation for fighting the good fight in rush-hour traffic. Put yourself in traffic and feel your foot alternating between the accelerator and the brakes.

You may ask about time order. Because you are taking the passage word by word or phrase by phrase, you would enact each as they arise, as if you had a video camera and were filming the action or association you are creating for each word or phrase in the order they come up. So, do not worry if there is some jumping around, because the key is to convert the word into an action in your mind so when asked to recall a question about the word or phrase, that action will pop up from your kinesthetic memory bank at any time, whether in order or not (unless it is a time order question—in which case refer to the strategies for remembering items in order).

Continue with the next phrase: "As he ran down the steps

of his apartment building...." Now imagine (feel) yourself running down the steps of an apartment building. What is the apartment building like? Imagine running around the building so your muscles can recall the steps you need to run or the direction to encircle it. Describe what is happening on your movie screen, theater production, or real-life experience that you created to go with that part of the passage.

Next, read "...heading towards his red sports car..." Pick a red sports car you would like to drive and feel the power of driving it. Think, "What do my muscles experience as I drive it and how does the power of the car surge through my body?"

"...he felt the humid air pressing in on him." Think, "What do my muscles do when they feel humidity?" Feel yourself grabbing a towel to wipe the sweat off your face.

"It was going to be another hot summer day in June." Think, "How would you kinesthetically portray to an audience a hot summer day in June? Would you feel yourself in a bathing suit running through lawn sprinklers to cool down? What comes to your mind when you think of June? Do you think of being at someone's birthday in June? Are you at a June wedding? If you think of vacationing in June, what would you do—go snorkeling or swimming? Whatever meaningful association you have for June use it. Remember, you want to hook this month into your prior knowledge, or whatever else is already in your head related to June. But don't use my examples—you must make up your own or it will not mean anything to you!

"Dave opened his car door..." Feel your arm muscles as you pull open a car door. Act it out in your mind.

"...tossed his brown attaché case onto the passenger seat..." Feel your muscles lift a heavy brown attaché case. Note that you are tossing it onto the passenger seat. Image yourself bouncing up and down in a passenger seat either of your own car or someone else's car you know.

"...and slid into the driver's side." Do this now. Slide into the driver's seat of your car. You will imagine yourself doing it.

"This was the only thing he looked forward to every morning, driving his new car along the freeway to his office." Experience racing that car along the highway.

"He looked forward to next week when he would begin a two-week vacation." To make an action out of "next week," imagine your arm muscles standing at a giant-size calendar and using the large motor muscles of the arm circling the next week. Then, kinesthetic people can experience packing a suitcase for a two-week vacation. To recall two weeks, the kinesthetic learner can think of fourteen days and mentally pack fourteen pairs of socks for their running shoes.

Now, focus on remembering the number "two"—what images come to your mind for "two?" Can you feel yourself *jump* off a diving board with your *two* feet? How about two basketball shots for a free throw opportunity? Find an association for the number two that is meaningful to you and experience it in your kinesthetic learning style.

"As he drove towards Interstate 72..." Another number—72. First you will experience yourself driving towards the interstate. You will experience an interstate you know in your own state. Now, work on the number 72. You can make any number of associations—what happened to you or what happened in the world in 1972? Or take it as 7 and 2. What action can you associate with 7 and what do you think of for number 2? Is there something that costs 72 dollars, someone you know who is 72 years old, some football player who wears number 72? Make the association happen on the interstate so you can connect these two together.

"...his mind raced along thinking about his holiday." Imagine yourself thinking about actions you will do on your own holiday as you drive along. Personalize it so you will remember it.

"Aruba sounds good with its dry air..." Now work on the name, Aruba." What action associations come to your mind? Think about what you would do if you went to Aruba. Take the word itself and think of something you already know that sounds like it or take the word apart and find smaller words that sound like those parts. For example, a-rub-a can be like a ruby—polish a red ruby. Or take the spelling instead of the sound—rub—a rub down on your back as you lay out on the beach. Or connect "arid" or dry to Aruba and say "arid Aruba." Experience arid, dry air. To remember arid and dry, imagine yourself as you pant for water as you hike along a hot desert. What do you experience yourself doing in the arid, dry air?

"... it's seventy-degree weather..." Another number—70 degrees. You can connect it with your interstate 72 image and subtract 2 to get 70, or you can think of another action association. Some examples that others have used are: some address with 70, someone who is 70, something that happened in 1970, or what you want to do when you are seventy? Experience that 70-degree weather.

"'... and its cool ocean breezes—a change from this stifling humidity,' he thought to himself." Now do something in cool ocean breezes. Are you surfing, swimming, sun bathing? Experience the stifling humidity. Do you experience yourself jumping in a cold shower to wash off that stickiness of the humidity? Image yourself experiencing these actions.

"A short ring from his cell phone startled him out of his daydream." Experience yourself talking about what you want to do as you talk to your friends on your hands-free cell phone. Experience yourself snap back to reality from your daydream as if parachuting down from a cloud and feeling a hard landing on earth.

Now, let us do a practice kinesthetic reading comprehension and memory test to see how much you remember of the story having made it in an action experience that happened to you in your mind. Answer the following questions, *without* looking back at the story. The answers are at the end of this section of this chapter, but no peeking or the point of this practice memory exercise will be lost!

1. Name who this story is about.
2. In what kind of home does he live?
3. What time of day does the story begin?
4. What is the weather like outdoors when the story begins?
5. What month of the year is it when the story begins?
6. Where is he going that morning?
7. Is he on time?
8. What kind of car does he own and what color is it?
9. What route will he take?
10. What was the only thing he looked forward to each morning?
11. Where is he thinking about going on vacation?
12. When is he going on his vacation?
13. What is the weather like in the place he is going for his vacation?
14. What is the temperature like in the place he is going for his vacation?
15. What startled him as he drives to work?

If you imaged the story in your kinesthetic Superlink learning style and brain style as I guided you through the reading, you should have found, as does everyone else who has successfully used this technique, that you were able to answer every question for which you made a strong action you were doing in your mind. If you missed any questions, analyze why. Most likely you missed a question because you did not make a strong enough action you felt yourself doing in your mind or you skipped it without imagining it. It is always fascinating to see that the movie scenes that people do not make are gone from their memory when they try to answer the questions, while the movie scenes they did make pop out as if they really experienced the event for themselves!

If you convert each detail of what you read and hear into this experiential event or action movie in your mind, you will be able to put into long-term kinesthetic memory everything you wish. You can do this kind of reading with everything you read, fiction or nonfiction. You can do this with the physical or digital texts, such as the daily newspaper, magazine articles, trade journals, memos, bulletins, interoffice communications, blogs, e-mail, faxes, website or social media sites. The same technique can work with a novel as well as with science material, technical reading, history, social sciences, health, textbooks in any content area subjects, medical books, training manuals for any field, and anything else you can think of.

The next question you may ask is, "Doesn't it take a long time to read this way?" The reply is, "no, it is actually quicker." It only seemed longer because you are just learning the technique and I had to "talk" you though this initial practice memory exercise to train you and model for you how to read or listen in this way. I was guiding you with a series of questions advising you on what to think about as you read, but you will take over from here and begin to ask yourself the questions as you read: "What am I doing now or experiencing myself doing now in my movie?" When you think this, it takes only a few seconds. As you practice this technique for several weeks, you will not need to ask the question anymore--you will automatically begin to experience the action as you read. After a few weeks or months, you will find that the moment you read the words, the action takes place. Soon, reading will be like a continual movie you are acting in playing in your head in which you are not even conscious of the words at all. You will actually read faster because you will be immediately experience the actions and you will move along continually without stopping at phrases anymore. Best of all, you will have increased and improved your memory to read and recall everything you choose!

Memory Improvement Exercise 2: Find something to read on the subject you have chosen to learn. Take two or three paragraphs and practice reading them as you did in the sample passage reading in this chapter. After each phrase, ask yourself what are you doing with your large motor muscles or what are you experiencing kinesthetically? Read the entire passage in that way. Then put the book down and see how many details you can recall, focusing on names, dates, places, and small facts. Practice reading in this kinesthetic way with all reading material from now on until you find you can mentally act out the movie automatically, the moment you scan the words.

Answers to questions on the Sample Practice Reading Comprehension and Memory Passage: "Dave":

1) Dave; 2) an apartment or apartment building; 3) morning; 4) humid, or hot and humid; 5) June; 6) to work; 7) no, he is late; 8) red sports car; 9) Interstate 72 or the freeway; 10) driving his car on the freeway (or to work); 11) Aruba; 12) next week; 13) dry air, cool ocean breezes, or seventy-degree weather; 14) seventy degrees; 15) a phone call.

Step 4: Keeping that Memory Active by Retrieving It and Using It

The next step is to make sure the information you read stays in your mind, as an active file, readily accessible at your fingertips, by deciding how often you need to use the information you learned and for what purposes. Think of it as having material immediately accessible on your computer's hard disk as opposed to putting it on flash sticks or thumb drives and filing them somewhere deep in your closet.

There may be certain types of information that are only needed for a one-time purpose. You may need to pass a test or exam and never need that information again. Suppose you took an art history course that was required for your fine arts degree. You do not want to go into art history, but you do want to be an artist. You need the information to pass the test for your degree, but you do not want to load your mind with dates when famous paintings were completed. Thus, you consciously decide to retain that data only so long as you need it to pass the examination and then let it go. You no longer want to work at keeping that memory active. Thus, you do not devote any more attention to it, and you do not use it or retrieve it anymore. Therefore, it is buried by newer, more relevant data that you need to learn.

Step four in training your memory involves making a conscious choice about which long-term memories you wish to keep in an active file and which ones you will allow to be buried in an inactive state. To keep a file active we need to use it and retrieve it periodically. You may not use the dates of the paintings ever again in your life so you let them go, but if you worked as a tour guide in an art museum, you would use that information again and again. It would become a part of you, and you could instantly bring it from memory, whenever you needed it. If we took a computer course and needed to use what we learned on our jobs every day, we would not want to forget the information after the final examination. By using the information daily, we strengthen the neural network or the interconnections that enable us to perform those functions. Retrieval becomes quicker and more automatic, for when we repeatedly use the information we made a conscious effort to learn; it becomes part of our long-term memory.

Step four requires you to decide how long you want to keep what you learned as an active long-term memory and when and how often you will need to use what you learned. Then, make a plan for retrieving and using it regularly. If you decide you need to use it for the one year in which you will be working at a particular job, then you need to spend time practicing using it, doing something with it, or retrieving it daily, weekly, or several times a week so it is fresh in your mind. Put it on your "to-do" list. As a kinesthetic learner, do something with it related to the material. This will keep the memory active. The more you use it, the more automatic retrieving this memory will become.

Exercise: Using the subject you are learning as an example to practice the kinesthetic techniques in this book, decide how long you want to retain the information as an active long-term memory. When and how often you will need to use what you learned? Make your personal plan for retrieving and using the material regularly.

What about Memorization?

Another kind of memory task is pure memorization, which involves recalling lists of facts and data. If you find you have to memorize information just to pass a test or exam, then you can also use your kinesthetic Superlink learning style and brain style to accomplish this task quickly. Try it with a list of data you need to remember. Practice the technique until it becomes automatic.

Take the data you are trying to learn and make action associations with something you already know. It can be a word that sounds like or is spelled like the word you need to remember. It may be a person or action that comes to your mind when you think of that word. You need to make up a movie or story in your mind connecting the new word on the list with the old word. The story should be vivid, humorous, imaginative, or far-out—something that will catch your attention and stay in your mind. You will need to enact the associations into a story in a different way based on your kinesthetic Superlink style.

The main difference between the left brain and right brain techniques is that left brain people will need to remember the list in order. The right brain people can make the associations without going in order unless this is required for a test or task; then the right brain people can use the left brain technique combined with their learning style.

Memorizing Data: Suppose you need to recall the following list of words: cat, house, moon, apple, football. Here is how you will use your kinesthetic Superlink brain and learning style to do it.

Right Brain: Remember the associations without putting them in order.

Left Brain: Remember them in linear order. Here is one way to do it: Take your hands and lay them palms down in front of you. Using your left hand first, count on your fingers, beginning with the pinkie, as follows: pinkie finger is one, ring finger is two, middle finger is three, pointer or index finger is four, and thumb is five. Now you will imagine that you are attaching each of the five words to each of your five fingers, in order, beginning with the word *cat*. You will do it according to your kinesthetic Superlink learning style technique below:

Kinesthetic Technique: You will need to act out the words: 1) You are a cat and are crawling around on the floor. Take hold of the owner's pinkie finger and pull him or her playfully to romp on the floor. 2. You are building a house and in your exercise room you hang ropes with large rings from which to swing. Experience yourself swinging from the rings that are shaped like the ring on your ring finger. 3. You are doing a handstand on the moon, balancing on your middle finger. 4. You are twirling an apple on your pointer finger and tossing it up and down in the air. 5. You catch a football with your thumb and then run to the goal line to make a touchdown. Now, when you flick each of your five fingers actions did you do for each? Do you remember all the words?

Mnemonics as a Memory Device for the Kinesthetic Superlink Learning Style and Brain Style

You can try another memory improvement technique, mnemonics, by using the first letter of each word to make either a new word or a sentence using words that begin with the same first letters as the words in the list. The left brain people will put the letters in order, while the right brain people can mix up the order to create other sentences or words.

The **kinesthetic people** will *stand up and write* the words in large print at a chalk board or white board, or will use big blocks or cut out shapes with the letters on them and move them around. Or they will experience themselves doing an action with the words in their minds.

For example, to remember the five words: *cat, house, moon, apple,* and *football,* here are a left brain and a right brain memory improvement technique:

Left brain people can put the words in order to make the nonsense word: *chmaf: c* for *cat; h* for *house; m* for *moon; a* for *apple;* and *f* for *football.* Or they can make a sentence from the first letter of each word: Can *he m*ake *a f*ire? Added to that can be the actual words as part of the story. Can he make a fire? Have the moon shining over the house, as the cat sitting, on a football, chews an apple by the fire.

Right brain people can mix-up the order in any way. Since the right side sees all the letters of a word simultaneously and does not put things in sequential order, it can remember them as effectively in any order it likes. For example: "cham(p)." Replace *f* with *p* and associate the *f* with the word *football:* He was the champ in football.

Another technique is to make a sentence with the first letters of each word arranged in any order: *My f*riend *has a* cat. You can then add the relevant words to this sentence to make a story: While you were sitting in your house, under a full moon, your friend came over with the cat, which was playing with a football and an apple.

The key to improve and increase your memory is to make action associations that are meaningful to you, that are out of the ordinary, and that tie the new words to the old words in some way.

Improving Memory by Creating a Story

Another technique is to connect all the words to make a unified story in which you play an active part. You will do one or a combination of the following based on your kinesthetic Superlink learning style and brain style: act out the story mentally. The following is an example: "You and your cat were taken from the house and sent up to the moon. You had apples to eat on the way. When you got to the moon you played football together and it was fun because you could bounce really high."

Improve Memory of Vocabulary Words in English or Other Languages:

Learning any field often requires understanding new terminology and vocabulary, so this section will be useful to improve memory in many situations. You can use this technique to learn and improve your memory of the meaning of new words, either English or other languages. Remember, the kinesthetic learners will do some action with the words.

English Vocabulary Words:
abase: to lower, humiliate
abashed: embarrassed, ashamed

Step 1: Take the word and find another word that looks or sounds like it and is already in your memory bank: Example: abase: sounds like *base*, something that is on the ground.

Step 2: Make up an action story connecting the word you already know with the meaning of the new word: for example, "I was so humiliated when I lost that I wanted to sink into the *base* or the ground."

Step 3: Connect the story with your kinesthetic Superlink learning style and brain style. You will be playing a basketball game and when you lose, you are humiliated and will fall down on the base, or floor.

When you see or hear the word *abase* in the story you created, the word will replay like a movie in your head and the concept of humiliation and lowering will come up as a movie scene, giving you its meaning.

Let's try the next word: abashed: ashamed. The word *abashed* sounds and looks like *bashed*. When you bashed into the wall because you weren't looking, you were ashamed. Act it out in your mind, and the word is yours.

Words in other languages: The same principle can be used for learning how to learn and improve your memory and vocabulary for words in different languages. For example: Here are steps if you want to remember the French word *maison,* which means "house."

Step 1: Think of a word that sounds like, looks like, or is similar to *maison*, or the parts of the word: May's son; my son; maize or corn; May sun.

Step 2: You will make up an action story connecting the association with the meaning of the word. Let's take "May sun." Link the hot May sun in the sky and their house. Come up with a sentence such as, "The May sunshine was beating down on my house, so I went outdoors to play golf."

Step 3: Connect the story with their Superlink learning style. Kinesthetic learners will act it out.

Let us try an example with a Spanish word *blanco*, which means "white" Connect *blanco* to a blank sheet of paper that is white. Now you have *blanco* as "white," but imagine an action with it. For example, "I am making a blanco paper airplane, or white paper airplane, and throwing it."

A Trained Memory Accelerates Learning

By improving your memory, you can learn something correctly the first time and cut down the wasted study time rereading and restudying the same material. You can accelerate your learning by training your memory using your kinesthetic Superlink learning style and brain style.

Chapter 7:
Applying What You Have Learned About Improving a Kinesthetic Learner's Memory and Learning

The knowledge you gained in this book about kinesthetic learning can empower you with the skill of knowing how to learn any subject quickly and to master it. To date, this is the current technology available to us. With each passing year, more research findings and newer technologies will provide us with still more ways to accelerate our learning. If you did the practice exercises, you would already have used these tools to work through one subject that you selected as a practice case.

To apply what you learned in this book, select a subject as you work through the activities. Also have a goal or purpose for learning that subject. Think about what that goal is. If you work through all these practice activities, you will be well on your way to mastering your subject by using the tools provided in the book. You can then apply this to learn other areas. Take a moment and list other areas that you would like to learn. Then, go through all the exercise pages in the book to complete your personal plan for learning each of these subjects.

Many people think of learning as a dead-end road. They

learn something and that is the end of it. Few people actually *use* what they learn. Many people take courses and never apply the material or skills they have learned to their lives. Twelve years of schooling, possibly sixteen or more if we go to training schools, colleges, or higher education, have conditioned us into taking courses, passing tests, and forgetting the material the following day. As a society, we have come to equate learning with passing tests and getting grades, diplomas, or certificates. However, the true nature of learning is a transformation into a better self, a higher self, a fully-developed self. As a by-product, we can put what we learned into the service of humanity at large and make the world a better place. Learning is a tool to help us achieve our goals and dreams.

If we are learning a skill for a current job or hobby, we are most likely going to apply what we learned on a regular basis. If we have learned a new subject unrelated to our current activities, the following are some examples of how we can apply these to everyday life:

Literature: Continue to read on your own; start a discussion group; keep a journal; and do your own writing.

Sports or dance: Find some friends or join a group to practice a sport or dance.

Using the Internet: Spend time daily "surfing" to locate websites related to your interests.

Carpentry: Start a small project, building something for your home or family or friends

Cooking: Invite friends over for a gourmet meal.

Marketing: Take a product your business produces and improve on marketing it.

Health: Set some personal health goals in the areas of diet, nutrition, fitness, or exercise; start a personal program for yourself or join a fitness club.

Quantum Physics: Find a laboratory to visit or work in, either part-time or as a volunteer so you can apply what you learned to research; join a book study group on the subject.

Learning is more than studying for a test. Having passed our examinations or performance assessments and proven our knowledge of a subject or skill, we do not want to have wasted all that time and let our knowledge fade away with disuse. True, there may be subjects we had to take for which we had no use. Focus instead on those subjects that you chose to study as part of your life's work, goals, interests, hobbies, or talents. The process of accelerated learning is complete when we use what we learned right away.

In the past, learners used to do tons of practice activities, yet did not recall the subject when they were assessed months later because they did not apply what they learned. When they used their knowledge and skills in everyday life the material stayed in their long-term memory. The final stage in accelerated learning is to use what you learned in your daily life.

Exercise: Think about a subject you select to learn as you work through this book. List all the ways that you can apply to your daily life what you gained from this book about the kinesthetic Superlink learning style and brain style for your personal transformation, to help others, or to transform the world.

APPENDIX

Kinesthetic Appendix: How to Use Your Kinesthetic Superlink Learning Style and Brain Style to Improve Memory, in Different Fields of Learning

As a kinesthetic learner embarks on one's lifelong learning plan, one may encounter a variety of fields that one must learn. This section provides sample applications of how to use your kinesthetic left or right brain Superlink learning style and brain style to improve memory to master different fields of learning. These sample applications provide examples to improve memory to apply what you learned about your kinesthetic Superlink and accelerated learning to master different subjects.

The sample applications are in the following fields: math, writing, technical reading (computer manuals), the sciences, sports, and vocational fields and hobbies. For each subject, adaptations for your kinesthetic Superlink learning style and brain style are provided giving you memory strategies to boost your brain power and use it to accelerate your learning in that field.

Application of the Kinesthetic Superlink Learning Style and Brain Style to Improve Memory for Learning How to Learn Math

Math is used in all segments of society. It is used for business, for home and personal use, for school and college courses in math, or use of math in other fields such as science, economics, history, computer science, health, nutrition, art, music, or vocational fields. We can use our kinesthetic Superlink learning style and brain style to improve memory for accelerating our ability to learn how to learn math. The following are some basic adaptations to use for learning any field of math using our kinesthetic Superlink.

Kinesthetic Left Brain: Physically act out story problem using concrete real-life examples in a game, simulation, or role-play in a step-by-step way and talk about it. Write the numbers in large size while standing up at a board or flipchart, and talk through the problem in a step-by-step way. Use sports or game equipment, physical exercise, or movement as a bonus for working out each problem to keep actively engaged while doing the math.

Kinesthetic Right Brain: Physically act out the story problem with concrete, real-life examples in a global way with the answer. Do several examples of the same type of problem with the answers so the right side of the brain can understand the pattern of how to do it. Use large manipulative materials to illustrate the problem. Write the numbers and the problem in large-size while standing up at a board or flipchart. Play sports, games, or do a physical activity while practicing the math problem. Keep the body physically engaged during the process of working the problems.

Application of the Kinesthetic Superlink Learning Style and Brain Style to Learn How to Learn and Improve Writing Skills

Good writing is essential for communication, whether it is for business, essays and research for schools and colleges, personal communication, or for technical writing for computer programs or instruction manuals. We can use our kinesthetic Superlink learning style and brain style to increase our memory to learn writing skills.

Planning the Outline for Left Brain Learners

Left Brain: Plan out the piece by making the left brain outline format of the "Evaluative Checklist for Good Writing" by standing up and writing the outline on a flip chart or white board. In your mind, visualize yourself doing the actions involved in each portion of the story. Physically act out or role play what you want to write about if it is possible. After writing the piece, mount the evaluative checklist for writing on a board. Stand up and read aloud your piece, using your large arm muscles to check off or put an action sticker for each item on the checklist that you have covered. Rewrite the piece to see that all components are covered.

Planning the Outline for Right Brain Learners

Right Brain: Draw a mind map of the piece as a plan before doing the actual writing. After writing the piece following the mind map, make the "Evaluative Checklist for Good Writing" into a mind map form of the points to go over to evaluate the piece to make sure all components are included.

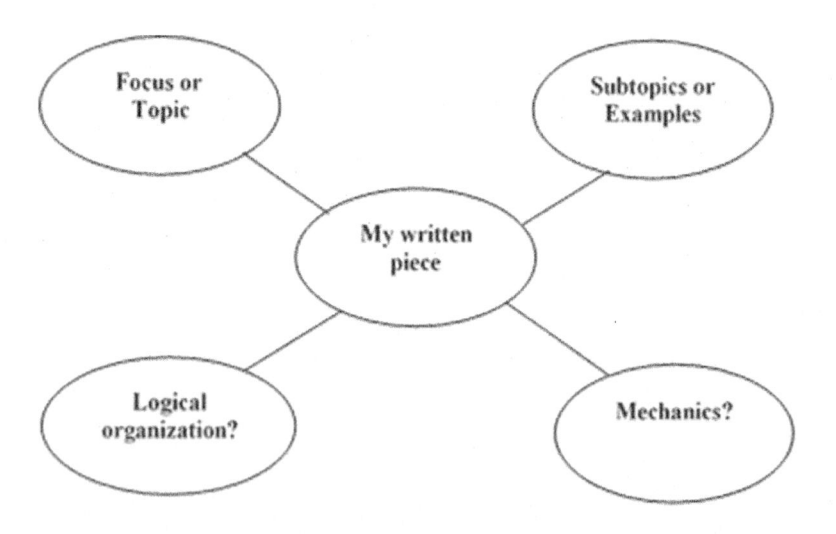

```
   ( Focus or  )              ( Subtopics or )
   (  Topic    )              (  Examples    )
         \                     /
          \                   /
           ( My written )
           (   piece    )
          /                   \
         /                     \
   (  Logical   )              ( Mechanics? )
   (organization?)
```

This format helps the right brain learner copy graphically what they need to include in a written piece.

Application of the Kinesthetic Superlink Learning Style and Brain Style to Improve Memory to Learn How to Learn Technical Reading

Driving the information highway or surfing the Internet requires ability in the field of technical reading. Technical reading has become an important area that does not receive much attention in reading programs. It is needed to read data on your computer screen, instructional manuals, computer manuals, and directions for using everyday technological equipment, such as cameras, microwaves, cars, assembling furniture, or installing a software program. Below are adaptations to help you use your kinesthetic Superlink learning style and brain style to improve memory to master technical reading.

Kinesthetic Left Brain: Physically do or perform the actions described in the reading in a step-by-step way as you read. Read while working on the actual equipment or tools. Make a large left brain outline on a flipchart or board as you read, while standing up. Talk through the steps aloud as you perform them. Wherever possible, relate the material to the actual performance of the task.

Kinesthetic Right Brain: Look over the material, focusing on the introduction and the conclusion and the main headings before reading. Look at any diagrams, pictures, or charts first.

As you go through the technical manual, make a large size mind map on a flip chart or large board while standing up, sketching out with pictures and key words the main points. Physically perform the task as you read for best results. You will probably want to jump right in and do it, and learn by trial and error. You can do so, but refer to the technical reading as a double check to make sure you are in the right direction.

Application of the Kinesthetic Superlink Learning Style and Brain Style to Increase Memory to Learn the Sciences

There are many fields of sciences, but there are certain common characteristics in learning each of them: reading research of others and experimenting by forming hypotheses and testing them using the scientific method. These processes can be adapted for the kinesthetic Superlink learning style and brain style so that any kinesthetic person can be successful in improving memory to learn the sciences.

Kinesthetic Left Brain: As you read scientific material, visualize yourself sequentially doing the actions described. If possible, physically perform the actions described in the reading in a step-by-step way as you read. Read while working on the actual science equipment. Plan your experiment by making a large left brain outline on a flipchart or board as you read, while standing up. Talk through the steps aloud as you perform them. Wherever possible, relate the material to the actual performance of the task. Keep a record of what you have done by making a large chart on a board while standing up. You will do well to work in a group setting, making it more active and lively.

Kinesthetic Right Brain: Look over the material, focusing on the introduction and the conclusion and the main headings before reading. Look at any diagrams, pictures, or charts first. As you go through the science readings, make a large size mind map on a flip chart or large board while standing up, sketching out with pictures and key words the main points. Draw or sketch out while standing up your plan for the experiment. Use color, symbols, and icons wherever possible. Do the experiment and record the results in a mind map on a flipchart, with sketches. You will probably want to jump right in and do it, and learn by trial and error. You can do so, but double check to make sure you are working in the right direction. Work in a group setting, making it more active and lively.

Application of the Kinesthetic Superlink Learning Style and Brain Style to Increase Memory to Learn Sports or Dancing

---

Some people seem to take naturally to sports or dance. They just seem to pick these up with natural ease. Sports and dance are other areas that can be best learned if adapted to one's natural style of learning. People with a kinesthetic Superlink learning style and brain style can increase memory to learn how to learn and master sports or dancing if instruction is compatible with the way their brain thinks. The following are adaptations so that people with a kinesthetic Superlink learning style and brain style can learn or improve in mastering sports and dancing.

Kinesthetic Left Brain: Join in with others who are performing the sport or dance and follow along in a step-by-step way. Have a coach guide you through it, giving you step-by-step verbal directions and carry it out as you listen. Your kinesthetic sense will get an automatic feel for the movements and it will come easily and naturally for you. You can pick it up just by working with others who are performing it in a step-by-step way.

Kinesthetic Right Brain: You will learn it by just jumping in and doing the sport or dance with others. Observe the entire process first so you have the big picture or overview. Then just get involved by doing it. Learning a sport or dance by doing it comes easily for you. By participating, you learn by trial and error. A coach can guide you where you need refinement. The action and movement of the sports and dance, and the fun of competition, makes this an easy area for you to master.

Application of the Kinesthetic Superlink Learning Style and Brain Style to Increase Memory to Learn Vocational Fields and Hobbies

There are numerous vocational fields and hobbies in which people are engaged for work and play. These involve learning a skill that needs to be performed. This area ranges encompasses construction, architecture, designing, landscaping, interior decoration, plumbing, electrical engineering, painting, wallpapering, gardening, agriculture, farming, carpentry, building airplanes, trucks, or cars, delivery, driving, trucking, shipping, sales, marketing, crafts, textiles, sewing, knitting, fashion designing, jewelry making, modeling, art, music, machine repairs, restaurant and food industry, entertainment, and numerous other fields. Learning any of these fields can become easy and quicker if the instruction is adapted to our Superlink learning styles and brain styles. The following are kinesthetic adaptations to increase memory to learn any vocational field or hobby through your kinesthetic Superlink learning style and brain style.

Kinesthetic Left Brain: Join in with others who are performing the task and follow along in a step-by-step way. Have a coach guide you through it, giving you step-by-step verbal directions and carry them out as you listen. Your kinesthetic sense will get an automatic feel for the job and it will come easily and naturally for you. You can pick it up just by working with others who are performing it in a step-by-step way.

Kinesthetic Right Brain: You will learn it by just jumping in and doing the task with others. Observe the entire process first so you have the big picture or overview. Then just get involved by doing it. Learning by doing comes easily for you. By participating, you learn by trial and error. A coach can guide you where you need refinement. The action and movement of a skill or task makes this easy for you to learn.

BONUS FOR READERS

How to Find Your Fasters Way of Learning: How to Take the Superlinks Learning Style Inventory Test: Linksman Learning Style Preference Assessment™ and Linksman Brain Hemispheric Preferences Assessment™

If you wish to take the Superlinks Learning Style and Brain Style Inventory, consisting of the Linksman Learning Style Preference Assessment™ and Linksman Brain Hemispheric Preference Assessments,™ a simple, quick online learning style and brain style assessment inventory that is automatically scored, giving instant results in a personalized report, you can go to any of the following three websites:

www.superlinkslearning.com, or
www.readinginstruction.com,
or www.keystoreadingsuccess.com

which is the accelerated program of K-12, college and adult reading, memory, note taking, study, and test-taking skills. The Superlinks test is the same whether taken through either of these 3 Internet sites. There is an English and Spanish version of the tests, with more languages in the works. The assessment on the Keys to Reading Success™ website also contains a pre-K, kindergarten, Grade 1 through Grade 12, college, and adult reading diagnostic test, instantly scored with a prescriptive reading plan to accelerate learning, plus lessons to improve reading comprehension, memory, study skills, phonics, fluency, vocabulary, and test-taking for reading in any content area subject through each of the brain's eight Superlinks learning styles and brain styles or your fastest way of learning. Lessons have adaptations for all Superlinks learning styles and brain hemispheric preference styles. It contains an entire reading comprehension, memory, study, and test-taking skills curriculum for any age, whether for pre-K, kindergarten, Grade 1 through Grade 12, college, or adult, in each of the Superlinks learning styles and brain hemispheric preference styles.

Once you take the Superlinks learning style and brain style test, you will get your results and a detailed report on how you learn the best, what materials you need, what is the best learning environment, what is the best learning strategies, and how you best communicate with others and want others to communicate with you.

Find Your and Other's Fastest and Best Way of Learning to Improve Memory, Reading Comprehension, and Learning

You can go to the website to get a license to take the online version of the Superlinks test. **Note:** Use the special discount code provided to the readers of this book *How to Quickly Improve Memory and Learning for Kinesthetic Left and Right*

Brain Superlink Learning Styles. The discount will give you access to the test at a nominal fee from the usual cost for the test. To access a license to take the test, go to:

http://www.superlinkslearning.com

and select from the Explore Learning Store: Superlinks to Accelerated Learning™ Assessment and enter the discount code: HTLAQ or contact info@keyslearning.com

If you are a teacher, parent, coach, trainer, sports coach, employer, or someone who wishes to have students, trainees, employees, athletes, or group members take the test, you can get bulk licenses at special rates by contacting info@keyslearning.com.

It will score the results for you instantly and automatically and give you an instant personalized report of your best Superlink. From there, go to the chapter that describes your Superlinks learning style and brain style to begin using the revolutionary brain-based approach for learning any subject—fast.

ABOUT THE AUTHOR:
RICKI LINKSMAN

Ricki Linksman is the author and developer of one of the fastest brain-based memory improvement, accelerated learning, learn to read, improve reading comprehension, and learn anything quickly program in the world today. She is the author of many books, including *How to Learn Anything Quickly: Quick, Easy Tips to Improve Memory, Reading, Comprehension, Test-Taking, and Learning through the Brain's Fastest Superlinks Learning Style*; *The Fine Line between ADHD and Kinesthetic Learners: 197 Kinesthetic Activities to Quickly Improve Reading, Memory, and Learning in Just 10 Weeks: The Ultimate Parent Handbook for ADHD, ADD, and Kinesthetic Learners*; *How to Improve Memory Quickly by Knowing Your Personal Memory Style: Quick, Easy Tips to Improve Memory through the Brain's Fastest Superlinks Memory and Learning Style*; *Your Child Can Be a Great Reader*; and *Solving Your Child's Reading Problems through Learning Styles*, featured in *Publisher's Weekly, Women's World, Family Life, Chicago Parent, Chicago Tribune, Los Angeles Parent, San Diego Parent*, the *Naperville Sun*, and the *Lisle Sun*. She has written numerous other books on accelerated learning and reading comprehension. Her newest one is *The Power of Mental Golf,* co-authored by Kerry R. Graham, LPGA Hall of Fame, Teaching and Club Professional Division and former president of LPGA, and Ricki Linksman, where Superlinks learning and brain styles can be used by golfers, golf professionals, and golf instructors and coaches to dramatically improve golf instruction and accelerate the speed of learning golf through a golfer's best way of learning.

Ricki Linksman is the founder-director of National Reading Diagnostics Institute, headquartered in Naperville, Illinois, near Chicago, a training institution to help people of all ages accelerate learning and improve their memory through Superlinks™ a system she developed using neuroscience and brain research, learning styles, and brain styles. Through Ricki Linksman's methods, people can improve their performance on their job and in their studies. By improving comprehension and memory of what they read, people can excel in any field. She runs a training institution in which trainers, sports and life coaches, instructors, administrators, employers, and teachers in any field can learn how to be more effective in training employees, students, and trainees.

She also directs a parent center in which she offers reading diagnostic testing and learning style and brain style inventory assessments to find one's fastest way of learning and remembering. Through diagnostic testing her methods include developing an individual prescriptive plan followed by coaching, teaching, and tutoring students from pre-K, kindergarten, Grades 1 through Grades 12, college, to adult learners. Students show dramatic improvement whether they are in regular education, special education, Title 1, remedial reading, have ADHD or ADD, are in bilingual or ESOL, ELL, ESL, or dual language programs, or who are gifted. She was the developer of one of the first parent involvement programs in the country, and was featured in Cendant and Davidson's Reading Blaster™ 9-12 popular software program as creating a "Parent Tips" guidebook, and was chosen as one of the best reading experts in the country to consult in the production of Cendant's *Learn to Read*™ software package. At National Reading Diagnostics Institute, parents are trained how to accelerate their children's or teens' memory and learning. Her Keys to Reading Success™ program includes parent involvement worksheets to help parents be more effective in providing homework help.

Ricki has been serving students in public and private schools throughout the country and around the world. Whenever she has set up the system of accelerated learning and accelerated reading in schools, those schools have raised test scores and achievement through her memory methods within less than one school year. Test scores raised include CTBS, SAT, ACT, and ISAT (Illinois State Achievement Test). Her memory improvement program has also been used to prepare students for career examinations in diverse fields, such as medicine and law.

Ricki Linksman is also the developer of *Keys to Reading Success*™ an Internet-based pre-K, kindergarten, grades 1 through 12, and college reading program to use accelerated learning and memory techniques and learning styles and brain hemispheric preference strategies to teach students to learn to read or improve reading within four to eight months or less. The average success rate is 88-99% of all K-12 students using the program rise 2-5 grade levels in reading in 6-8 months, including students in regular education, special education, ELL, ESL, ESOL, bi-lingual and dual language, Title 1 or Remedial Reading, and gifted programs (and those with ADD or ADHD). Rusty Acree, a retired veteran and current football referee, of Richmond, Virginia, is one of many parents and grandparents who have seen the effectiveness of the program on his grandson. His grandson, who had been previously labeled with ADHD, had been left back in kindergarten for two years, yet still could neither recognize the letters of the alphabet nor read a word. When he was diagnosed by Ricki as a kinesthetic right brain learner and was taught how to read through his kinesthetic right brain Superlinks style he was able to learn the letters of the alphabet and could read his first book ever within 2 days. Rusty Acree who continued to see the phenomenal growth of his grandson over the next year to get to grade level in reading has called Ricki Linksman, "The Michael Jordan of Reading."

Ricki developed the *Superlinks to Accelerated Learning*™ program with its *Linksman Learning Style Preference Assessment and Brain Hemispheric Preference Assessment*™ used to discover a person's best memory Superlink (learning style and brain style) to accelerate learning.

Her programs Keys to Reading Success™ and Superlinks to Accelerated Learning™ were selected by a foundation, the "Cotchery Foundation," started by New York Jets football running back, Jericho Cotchery and his wife Mercedes Cotchery, to assist an elementary school in North Carolina raise its reading scores and is featured on the Cotchery Foundation website.

Her award-winning phonics program has been selected for use as the phonics curriculum used by Huntington™ Learning Centers throughout the country. Other companies that have used her Superlinks to Accelerated Learning™ programs include Kaplan On-line University; MFS Investment Management, Boston, a large Massachusetts financial institution who used Ricki Linksman's accelerated learning techniques to help trainers teach clients about mutual funds sales; and by one of the largest technology company in the world.

Ricki Linksman created a phonics game program specially designed for kinesthetic and tactile learners, but can be used with visual and auditory learners also, including those with a right brain or left brain preference, called Off the Wall Phonics™. It allows students to learn to master and remember every phonics patterns in the English language to move someone from beginning reading to college-level word reading ability within 10 game levels, of 10 games each. If followed, any student can raise their word-reading level, which can help their reading comprehension, by playing one game level per week for ten weeks, and studies have proven the average raise in word-reading level to be two to five grade levels in reading in that time.

A university football team used Keys to Reading Success™ and Superlinks to Accelerated Learning™ to improve football performance through learning and memory styles and brain styles, helping them to their first winning season. It dramatically changed the way football coaches taught the football play book to the athletes.

She has worked as a consultant to golf instructors to improve teaching of golf through Superlinks to Accelerated Learning™ learning styles. She was a consultant to a former White Sox baseball player on product development of a pitching aid to improve pitching skills using Superlinks to Accelerated Learning™ As a trainer of trainers she has improved the effectiveness of trainers to help them reach all participants of different learning styles.

Many schools and educational institutions in South Africa from elementary school to a college, including Learning

Identity, Reading Identity, Clifton Preparatory School, Hamilton School, Oasis Preparatory School, and Hilton College have adopted Keys to Reading Success and Superlinks to Accelerated Learning to improve memory and reading.

Ricki works as a consultant to businesses, companies, and educational institutions to help people accelerate and improve memory and learning in any field. She has done trainings for college professors and instructors at colleges and universities. She has also done volunteer work training tutors for Literacy Volunteers for America. She trained facilitators for youth outreach programs sponsored by a local police station and worked with students from DCFS (Department of Children and Family Services). She has also served as a reading expert for a pro-bono court case for a major Chicago law firm. Public schools call on Ricki Linksman's expertise on case study teams for students.

She has run Administrator Academies in Illinois on District Reading Improvement, training superintendents and principals in steps to improve their district reading programs and scores. She has been one of the trainers for Illinois's ISAT (Illinois State Achievement Test) reading and writing tests and has trained teachers in how to raise test scores on this state test. She was one of Illinois's state validators for the Right to Reading Initiative. She has presented memory and learning strategies to many Regional Offices of Education to train teachers and administrators from many school districts in these methods.

She gives seminars and workshops, appears at booksignings, and speaks at conferences. She has presented her memory improvement and reading programs to tens of thousands of teachers across the country. She works as a consultant and trainer for public school districts and schools in accelerated learning techniques, raising district reading scores, and improving student achievement. She received a certificate of merit from the IASCD (Illinois Association for Supervision and Curriculum) 1999 Winn's Research Award for "Maximizing School Reading Scores."

She receives thousands of letters and emails from teachers, administrators, parents, college professors, consultants, and students from all over the world who have read her books and write to her for advice on improving memory, reading, and learning performance. Her works are cited on numerous Internet sites listing excellent resources for parents and teachers, including *Conde Nast*.

She has taught graduate education courses in reading, and another on inclusion: differentiated learning to teach to all learners through learning styles. Specializing in accelerated learning and memory improvement with application to reading, she has taught these techniques to students of all ages and to adults.

For parents and teachers, she has numerous books, eBooks, courses, online eCourses, podcasts, webinars, teleseminars, coaching, and consulting to accelerate learning for all types of learners, including kinesthetic, tactile, auditory, visual, with either a right brain or left brain preference. These materials have helped children and teens from pre-K, kindergarten, grade 1-12, and college, whether in regular education, special education, gifted, ESOL, ELL, ESL, bi-lingual or dual language, or Title 1 or Reading Remedial programs, or those who have ADHD or ADD.

CONTACT INFORMATION

Ricki Linksman can be contacted at:
National Reading Diagnostics Institute and Keys Learning,
Naperville, Illinois;

Email: info@keyslearning.com

Web sites:
http://www.readinginstruction.com
http://www.keyslearning.com
http://www.keystoreadingsuccess.com
http://www.superlinkslearning.com
http://www.nationalreadingdiagnosticsinstitute.com
http://www.offthewallphonics.com

A Special Gift for Readers

The author has a special gift for readers of this book, *How to Quickly Improve Memory and Learning for Kinesthetic Left and Right Brain Superlinks Learning Styles and ADHD*. If you would like to find your Superlinks learning style and brain hemispheric preference style, or that of your family, friends, and others, as a special reader of *How to Quickly Improve Memory and Learning for Kinesthetic Left and Right Brain Superlinks Learning Styles and ADHD*, here is your special discount code to access the test at a significant discount. Go to: http://www.readinginstructiom.com and from the Explore Learning Store, select Superlinks to Accelerated Learning™ Assessment and enter the discount code: HTLAQ

Note: When you get to the order page, scroll down to enter your discount code where the discounted price will appear. After taking the test, it will instantly be scored and give you a personalized report on your best Superlink learning style and brain style with tips on how to learn anything quickly. You can return to the matching chapter in this book or read one of the other books by Ricki Linksman in this series focused on your Superlink style to read about how you can learn quickly through your Superlinks learning style and brain style and improve your own or others' memory, reading, comprehension, note taking, study, test-taking skills, and learning. Enjoy the rewards of personal transformation!

For readers who enjoyed this book and feel it can help others, please visit amazon.com or other online sites if you want to write a review of how you enjoyed the book so that other struggling parents and teachers can help their child or students also go from pain and frustration to success.

Printed in Great Britain
by Amazon